THE
DIABETIC'S
BOOK

Also by June Biermann and Barbara Toohey

The Peripatetic Diabetic
The Diabetic's Sports and Exercise Book
The Diabetic's Total Health Book
The Diabetic Woman (with Lois Jovanovic-Peterson, M.D.)
The Diabetic Man (with Peter Lodewick, M.D.)
Psyching Out Diabetes (with Richard R. Rubin, Ph.D.)
Diabetes Type II and What to Do
(with Virginia Valentine, R.N., C.D.E.)

THE DIABETIC'S BOOK

All Your Questions Answered

JUNE BIERMANN
and
BARBARA TOOHEY

A Jeremy P. Tarcher/Putnam Book
published by G. P. Putnam's Sons
New York

Most Tarcher/Putnam books are available at special quantity discounts for bulk purchases for sales promotions, premiums, fund-raising, and educational needs. Special books, or book excerpts, can also be created to fit specific needs.
For details, write or telephone Special Markets, Putnam Publishing Group, 200 Madison Avenue, New York, NY 10016. (212) 951-8891.

A Jeremy P. Tarcher/Putnam Book
Published by G. P. Putnam's Sons
Publishers Since 1838
200 Madison Avenue
New York, NY 10016

Library of Congress Cataloging-in-Publication Data

Biermann, June.
The diabetic's book : all your questions answered / June Biermann and Barbara Toohey.—3rd rev. and expanded ed.
p.   cm.
"A Jeremy P. Tarcher/Putnam book."
Includes bibliographical references and index.
ISBN 0-87477-773-9 (pbk.)
1. Diabetes—Miscellanea.   I. Toohey, Barbara.   II. Title.
RC660.B459   1994   93-33777 CIP
616.4 ' 62—dc20

Printed in the United States of America
9   10

This book is printed on acid-free paper.

To Jackie Tippen,
who over the last thirty-three years
has given us the two greatest gifts:
love and work.

Contents

. . . .

All things are difficult
before they are easy.

—THOMAS FULLER, 1608–1661
Gnomologia No. 560

Foreword

. . . .

An old Talmudic saying goes "All beginnings are difficult." This couldn't be more true for persons with diabetes. To begin life over as a diabetic person is not only difficult but slightly short of impossible. Receiving the diagnosis of diabetes has nearly the same jolt as seeing your whole life—your inner house—collapse after an earthquake or hurricane.

The Diabetic's Book: All Your Questions Answered can be your guide to that new beginning. June and Barbara will lead you through the rebuilding and healing process with sound advice, knowledge, and wisdom gained over many years. They take the guilt out of "getting" the disease. It is hard to move forward when fear, anxiety, and anger are all pushing you back. Diabetes self-care necessitates information, skill, and concentration. This book provides it all.

Let me tell you why I feel so strongly about this tome.

First, it truly answers all your questions, as the title suggests. I know of few other books on diabetes that contain the wealth of information you will find here. The advice and facts are not only up-to-date but are substantiated by an extensive literature review and the secondary opinions of many leading experts in the field of diabetes self-care. June and Barbara also give you their own firsthand experiences and those of many other real people who live with diabetes day in and day out.

Second, this book teaches you the basic language of diabetes in a clear and straightforward manner. Each and every time a medical term is used, it is explained and defined. This is no small feat.

One of the worst complications of diabetes is actually the misunderstandings that frequently occur between diabetic patients and their health-care team. Thus, your new language skill will mean that the important communication between you and your doctor and dietician can begin.

Third, this work speaks to every diabetic, regardless of whether you are Type I or Type II (you will learn the difference in the first section), young or old, in control or out of control. I am particularly pleased with the coverage June and Barbara have provided for the person with Type II diabetes who is so often forgotten in other books on diabetes. In the past, Type II diabetes was thought to be a mild disorder that did not demand attention to blood glucose control. Today, we now know that Type II diabetes needs the full respect that Type I diabetes always had. Those of you with Type II diabetes need to keep your blood glucose levels as near to normal as possible to avoid the complications of diabetes. To achieve this goal, the Type II diabetic must adhere to diet, medication, exercise, and blood-sugar monitoring. This change in the philosophy of Type II diabetes treatment and self-care is clearly explained and beautifully chronicled by June and Barbara.

Fourth, there is a level of detail in this book that is unmatched in other beginner diabetes manuals. In every section, Barbara and June provide tiny gems of information that one generally does not find elsewhere. From diet tips to exercise hints to insulin injection equipment to advice for parents and families, you will find dozens of ideas that can truly make life easier for all involved.

From their suggestions, I learned to watch business trends for the latest breakthrough developments in diabetes control and treatment. Barbara and June are so right about this. After all, it only makes sense that we will learn about new discoveries and inventions in the pages of *The Wall Street Journal* and other business magazines before new diabetes products hit the market. By staying abreast of the business news, every diabetic person can follow the research done at dozens of companies and thereby feel a bit more hopeful that a cure is on the way.

Lastly, and perhaps most important, this book will motivate you to make the necessary changes in your life to live well with diabetes. As you read these pages, I am sure you will feel, as I did, that you are in good hands and that you have been truly understood. Through their own experiences with diabetes, Barbara and June know the ins and outs of depression, frustration, and fear. They write sensitively about what every diabetic person and concerned family member goes through, and they teach you how to have a sense of humor about it. It is easier to laugh when you know you are not alone, and diabetes is so much more tolerable to live with when you can laugh about dietary restrictions, injections, blood tests, mood swings, and annoying itches. June and Barbara will almost make you feel sorry for persons who do not have diabetes!

You will also find that this book can motivate your family and friends to a new beginning as well. The section addressed to them is worth the price of the book alone. Not only will they start to understand your diabetes, but they will gain a new sense of themselves and the role they can play in helping you to live a full and satisfied life rather than, as often happens, making "your" problem "their" problem.

When you have finished reading these pages, I am sure you will agree with my sentiments about this wonderful book. Thank you, June and Barbara. I enjoyed, I learned, I identified with all you have to offer here. Bravo for your new edition of *The Diabetic's Book*. All my questions *were* answered.

Lois Jovanovic-Peterson, M.D.
Senior Scientist, Sansum Medical Research Foundation,
Santa Barbara, California
Clinical Professor of Medicine,
University of Southern California,
Los Angeles

Introduction

· ·

Although this book is intended for anyone involved with diabetes—whether a newly diagnosed or experienced diabetic, a family member or friend, or a diabetes health professional—it is aimed primarily at beginners.

Why beginners? For two reasons. The first was born one day when the June half of our writing team was emerging from her dentist's office. The door to a neighboring internist's office opened and a man came out. He was clutching a copy of the American Diabetes Association's approved diet, *Exchange Lists for Meal Planning.*

The man had obviously just been given *the news,* because in ninety-six-point headlines his face was printed with confusion, fear, and despair. June could read these emotions easily because they were the same ones she'd seen in the mirror on her own D (for *diagnosis*) day. While writing this book, we've kept this man's face before us. Our goal has been to change his expression—and that of all newly diagnosed diabetics—to one of understanding, courage, and hope.

The second reason for aiming this book at beginners is based on the Zen theory of the expert's mind versus the beginner's mind. Since the expert's mind thinks it knows everything, it is closed to new ideas. It knows what *can't* be done. It thinks in terms of limitations. The beginner's mind, on the other hand, is still open. To the beginner all things are possible. Not even the sky is the limit.

We hope that this book will help all of you—no matter how many years you've had diabetes or have worked in the field of diabetes—to become beginners again.

1

THE DIABETICIZATION OF AMERICA

Lonely and lost though you may feel at the time of diagnosis, you are not alone in your diabetes. In the twelve years since the original publication of *The Diabetic's Book,* America has been what you might call "diabeticized." The estimated number of diagnosed diabetics has risen from 10 million to over 14 million, and there could be an equal number out there undiagnosed. As the population ages and longevity increases, the incidence of diabetes correspondingly goes up. Every year 750,000 new cases are diagnosed. Today, almost 18 percent of the population between the ages of sixty-five and seventy-four has diabetes, and this number is likely to double in the next twenty-five years. The cost of diabetes care now consumes 5 percent of the nation's health expenditures—$40 billion a year!

As a result of the recognition of diabetes as a burgeoning health problem and good old American free-enterprise desire for a chunk of the diabetes dollar, new products and therapies to make diabetes self-care easier and more effective are constantly being developed and improved.

Now instead of two blood-sugar meters, there are over a dozen—all smaller, faster, and much easier to use than ever before. Instead of one automatic insulin injector, there are five. Insulin infusion pumps have shrunk to the size of a pack of cards, and formerly complex jet injectors are now simple enough for children to operate.

But the diabeticization of America is not just having an impact on people with diabetes. Because of dramatic increases in medical costs for all Americans, there's a newfound interest across the country in following a healthy life-style. Self-care and preventive maintenance, long the cornerstones of a successful diabetes regimen, have become the recommended way of life for everyone. No, you are definitely not alone.

For example, you are not alone in your diet. The American way of eating has been thoroughly diabeticized. The diabetic diet, which people with diabetes used to consider strange and difficult to impose on the rest of the family, is now recognized as the ideal diet for everyone. It's identical to the one endorsed by the American Heart Association, the American Cancer Society, the Surgeon General, and most reputable weight-loss programs. New sugarfree, low-fat, high-fiber, low-sodium foods have appeared on the market to make it not only convenient to follow that diet but a pleasure as well.

All in all, thanks to diabeticization, things are very much better now than they were back in 1967, when June was diagnosed. Although it was not the worst of times, it was certainly not the best of times. Practical help for those with diabetes ranged between scarce and nonexistent. The now active, 7,000-member American Association of Diabetes Educators didn't even exist. The available diabetes books were ponderous and discouraging and written in boring, incomprehensible medical language. Those greatest tools for keeping your blood sugar under control—home blood-sugar-testing meters—hadn't been invented. People with diabetes were condemned to use inaccurate, awkward, and unesthetic urine tests. Blood-sugar tests were given monthly or quarterly, or even in some cases annually, in the doctor's office.

Because of this lack of help, information, and effective technology, we started devoting ourselves to finding ways to cope successfully with diabetes without becoming a slave to it and giving up all joys and excitements.

Using June as a guinea pig, we constantly checked out new angles of attack, seeing just how far we could push the envelope of diabetes. In conversations after our talks at diabetes associations, and in correspondence with hundreds of other diabetic people and health professionals who shared our good-life goals, we continued to learn more. We shared this newfound, ever-expanding and changing store of information and experiences in ten previous books on diabetes—including the two previous editions of this one.

Because *The Diabetic's Book* is our most basic and accessible book on diabetes, and because it has been used as a teaching text in many diabetes education programs, it has been read by more people than any of our other books on the subject. Over 100,000 copies are out there somewhere in Diabetesland. It has made us happy to be able to reach and, we hope, *teach* so many of those involved with diabetes. But a cloud slips over this happiness when we realize that a lot of the material from the last edition has already become out-of-date.

You'd think that in only three years not enough of significance in the field of diabetes could happen to warrant a third edition. But, believe us, it has! Nothing makes us more jubilant than to be able to tell you that so many changes for the better and so many breakthroughs have come about in this three-year period that this rewrite is mandatory. We don't want any of you to miss out on the new knowledge and therapies to make your life easier, happier, healthier, and *longer.* You'll find it all in this newly revised edition.

The highlights include:

- A new understanding of and expanded information for the neglected majority—the 90 percent of people with diabetes who are classified as Type II (non-insulin-dependent).

- Results of the ten-year Diabetes Control and Complications Trial (DCCT) that gave scientific proof of what we've believed and preached all along: good control can prevent—and in some cases reverse—diabetes complications.

- New forms and combinations of insulin and new methods of delivering it.

- The new FDA food pyramid and its relationship to diabetes meal planning.

- Demystification of the so-called diabetic diet.

- A complete update on equipment and instruments for diabetes home care.

- More help in purchasing supplies and making smart consumer decisions.

- Your benefits and protections under the 1990 Americans with Disabilities Act.

- The latest information on health insurance coverage.

- Practical advice in conquering negative emotions associated with diabetes.

- Expanded help for families and friends of people with diabetes.

- An updated bibliography of the best and brightest books on diabetes.

■ A complete new section on healthy and permanent weight-loss.

All in all, if you had to become diabetic, this is the best time in the history of the world for it to happen. Never before has it been so possible to keep your blood sugar in the normal range, to avoid (or reverse) the feared complications of diabetes, and to enjoy life as it was meant to be enjoyed. With this book we want you to learn how to live better with diabetes and *through* diabetes.

June Biermann
Barbara Toohey
Van Nuys, California
August 1993

Something for Everyone

. . . .

The old saying "You can't see the forest for the trees" is, like many such sayings, very true. Sometimes you're so close to the individual aspects of a problem, you can't see the whole picture. And not seeing the whole picture may prevent you from gaining the perspective necessary to attain overall control of the situation.

Therefore, before we launch into the specifics of how to take care of yourself as an insulin-taking or non-insulin-taking diabetic, or how to master the emotional aspects of the disease and manage your daily life, or how to offer the best support possible for your diabetic family member or friend, we'll take a look at the big picture of diabetes. This is what everyone needs to know. You'll find that once you see the forest of diabetes, you'll find it easier to get out of the woods.

DIABETES AND CONTROL

What is diabetes?

Diabetes is a physical problem that causes you to have too much sugar in your blood. The medical name for it is *diabetes mellitus.* The first word, *diabetes,* is from Greek and means "to run through a siphon." The second word, *mellitus,* is from Latin, and means "honey." The two words together are usually translated "sweet

7

water siphon." (In case you don't speak Greek and Latin, *diabetes mellitus* is pronounced *dye-uh-beet-ease mell-uh-tus.*) The doctors in ancient times called it that because they noticed that diabetics urinated a great deal and that their urine tasted sweet. Yes, *tasted* sweet. In those days the only way a doctor could test urine was by tasting it. (And doctors today won't even make house calls!)

Diabetes can be broken down into Type I, also called IDDM (*i*nsulin *d*ependent *d*iabetes *m*ellitus) and Type II or NIDDM (*n*on-*i*nsulin *d*ependent *d*iabetes *m*ellitus). Type I is the newer term for what used to be called juvenile-onset diabetes, because it occurs most frequently in people under the age of twenty. In actuality, Type I diabetes also affects people over twenty. For instance, June got diabetes as an adult in her forties, but she has to take insulin. Sometimes people like her are referred to as Type I ½ or Type II-D (for deficient). Her pancreas still produces some insulin, but not enough, while in true Type I's the pancreas produces no insulin at all.

Type II is the current term for what used to be called adult-onset diabetes. We now know that Type II diabetes is not limited to people over forty, as used to be thought, but that it occurs in teen-agers and even in some children. According to Stanley Mirsky, M.D., author of *Controlling Diabetes the Easy Way,* about 5 percent of Type II's are under twenty years of age.

Type I and Type II diabetes have such a number of differences that some experts theorize that they are actually two different diseases. But with both types there is the problem of too much sugar in the blood.

There is also a kind of diabetes that has nothing to do with blood sugar. It's called *diabetes insipidus,* and it is a problem of the hypothalamus rather than the pancreas. The hypothalamus produces an antidiuretic hormone that limits the formation of urine in the kidneys. When something (tumor, infection, or injury) damages the hypothalamus, interfering with the production of the hormone, excessive urination (along with excessive water drinking) is the result. Diabetes insipidus is sometimes called "water diabetes" to differentiate it from "sugar diabetes."

Diabetes insipidus can be hereditary and, like diabetes mellitus, can be controlled by the use of a hormone.

Why is there too much sugar in the blood?

The cells of the body run on a fuel called *glucose*. This is the sugar that the body manufactures from the food we eat. Glucose is carried to the cells in the bloodstream, but if you have diabetes it cannot be absorbed because the cells are locked up tighter than a Manhattan apartment. Glucose can't get into a cell without a key. That key is *insulin*. Insulin is a hormone that comes from a gland called the pancreas. The particular cells of the pancreas that produce insulin are the beta cells.

In Type I diabetes the beta cells have been totally destroyed and make no insulin, or have been partially destroyed and don't make enough insulin (Type I ½). That is to say, all or some of the insulin keys are missing so they can't let the sugar into the cells. Such people will need to inject insulin, which we will explain later.

In Type II diabetes, the beta cells are still there perking along, manufacturing plenty of insulin keys, but either the cells in the bloodstream don't have enough locks (called insulin receptors) for the insulin key to fit in, or something is keeping the locks from working. (This is called insulin resistance or insulin insensitivity.) These people will need to modify their diet, lose weight, and make other changes to control their diabetes. We will also explain this treatment shortly.

In both cases, the result is that sugar is left in the bloodstream, causing high blood sugar.

There is a convenient test doctors use to determine whether a diabetic still makes any insulin and roughly how much. It is called a C-peptide test and is a blood test ordinarily taken after overnight fasting and before breakfast. The more insulin your body makes, the higher your C-peptide level. The level of blood-serum C-peptide is usually zero in Type I diabetics. In Type II's it can be within or above the normal range.

What's wrong with having high blood sugar?

High blood sugar is an indication that your body is getting little or no fuel. In desperation it begins to convert its own fat and muscle into fuel. This is like chopping down the walls of your house to get wood to burn in your fireplace. If you keep that up, soon you have no house left.

But that's not even the worst of it. When the body burns itself for fuel, excess *ketones* (substances that are formed during the digestion of fat) are given off. These excess ketones can poison the body. This poisoning—called *ketoacidosis*—can lead to death. You may remember the television program about the California boy Wesley Parker, whose father threw away his insulin because a faith healer had "cured" the boy's disease. Within three days Wesley was dead from ketoacidosis.

There is also something else wrong with having high blood sugar. Let's say you have *some* insulin that's working—either insulin you've injected or insulin you've produced in your own pancreas—but you don't have enough. Or say you have plenty of insulin but it's not able to get the sugar into the cells. Then, while you won't use up your own body as fuel and you won't be poisoning yourself with ketones, you still have too much sugar flowing through your bloodstream. That's not good, because this situation brings about long-range diabetes complications like blindness, nerve damage, kidney failure, and gangrene of the feet.

What caused me to get diabetes?

Researchers have been puzzling over the answer to this question for decades. They have more leads now than ever before but still no definitive answer. We'll summarize what is known, and you can apply the information to yourself.

First, diabetes runs in families; so whether you got it as a child or later in life, you still had to have some genes that predisposed you to it. The two different types of diabetes are caused by different genes. Type I is much less hereditary than Type II. Second, diabetes favors certain ethnic groups: the incidence in Blacks, Hispanics, and Native Americans is over twice as great as in the Anglo population.

If you got Type I diabetes as a child (the commonest age to be diagnosed is around twelve) recent studies show that a virus related to the mumps, measles, or a similar infection might have attacked the insulin-producing beta cells of your pancreas. This triggered an immune response, so that your body's own immune system continued the destruction until after several years your insulin-producing capability was totally gone and you had diabetes. A recent study suggested that drinking cow's milk as an infant might trigger this same response. Scientists also suspect a possible environmental factor in childhood diabetes, since the highest incidence occurs in cold climates and more cases are diagnosed in winter than in summer.

For those diagnosed in midlife or later, the Type II's, more than one genetic defect is responsible. This form of diabetes develops slowly over a fifteen-to-twenty-year period. The number-one factor influencing the appearance of diabetes is excess weight. Some 80 to 85 percent of those diagnosed are overweight. Another influence is aging and a general slowing of body functions. More cases of diabetes are diagnosed after the age of sixty than at any other time of life.

Oddly, physicians have also discovered a special form of Type II diabetes that affects children and young people under the age of twenty-five. This is called MODY (maturity-onset diabetes of the young). Like adults, the children diagnosed with MODY are usually very overweight.

Overproduction of certain hormones—growth hormone from the pituitary, thyroid hormone, epinephrine, cortisone, and glucagon—makes the body's insulin less effective and can also bring on diabetes.

Pregnancy, which makes additional demands on the body, can cause diabetes to develop. In fact, some women show diabetes symptoms during pregnancy but their symptoms disappear after the baby is delivered. (This is called gestational diabetes.) Mary Tyler Moore wasn't that lucky. Her diabetes was diagnosed shortly after a miscarriage, and from then on she has been insulin-dependent.

Surgery or a major illness can activate diabetes. June became diabetic not long after a hysterectomy.

Many people have the mistaken idea that they can get diabetes from eating too much sugar. (As we said, diabetes is sometimes called "sugar diabetes," which adds to the confusion.) Diabetes can't be caused by eating too much sugar, except when your diabetes was triggered by overweight and you became overweight partly from overloading on sugar. But even in that case, it wasn't specifically the sugar that was to blame. Diabetes could have developed if you ate too much of anything and gained weight. The culprit is more likely the fat in your diet.

Why didn't I have any symptoms of diabetes when my case was diagnosed?

You were one of the thousands of hidden diabetics—people who have diabetes and don't realize it. You're one of the smart (or lucky) ones. You caught diabetes early, before it had done any real damage.

If you neglect your diabetes in the future, you may begin to experience the classic symptoms of the acute stages of diabetes: excessive urination and thirst, increased appetite, rapid loss of weight, irritability, weakness, fatigue, nausea, and vomiting. These indicate ketoacidosis, which if untreated will lead to coma and ultimately death. These are the symptoms that usually strike children and adolescents suddenly.

Most people who get Type II diabetes after the age of twenty have a different set of symptoms, though they may also have any of the above. Generally, the warning signals are drowsiness, itching, blurred vision, tingling and numbness in the feet, fatigue, skin infections, and slow healing. Type II diabetics often have two additional clues that diabetes may be in the offing: they are overweight, and they have a family history of diabetes.

Can diabetes be cured?

We're glad you didn't ask, "When will it be cured?" We're cured of making predictions because we've made so many in the past that didn't come true. For example, in the previous edition of this book, on the subject of beta-cell transplants, we quoted an eminent diabetologist who said, "The process has been patented and could be available as early as 1992." Look at your calendar.

But can it be cured? Of course. All things are possible and even probable. In fact, in a sense, some people have already been cured—

the hard way. Back in 1972 we met Mary Ellen Baran, who had had diabetes for twenty-three years. She was given a pancreas transplant and as a result became an instant nondiabetic.

We had breakfast with her and watched in amazement as she relished her pancakes and syrup. She confessed that "within three months of leaving the hospital, I had tested every dessert known and gained fifteen pounds." Fortunately, she soon got a grip on her new freedom, got her weight back to normal, and began eating more like the way she had before the operation. Believe it or not, she said she ended up eating *less* refined sugar than she had before her "cure."

In the ensuing years over 2,000 people throughout the world have received pancreas transplants with a success rate of between 40 and 80 percent. The transplants have been performed mainly on those who have had a kidney transplant and are already taking immunosuppressive drugs to keep the kidney from being rejected, since the same drugs will keep the pancreas from being rejected.

Since only those with kidney transplants have been cured so far, what is being done toward a cure for everyone else? The main focus of scientific effort now is not in transplanting entire pancreases (actually, as you might guess, there are very few of these available), but in implanting only beta cells to secrete the missing insulin. Beta cells can be injected from a syringe and will work if they can be protected from rejection by the body's immune system.

One of the new techniques for shielding the cells is to encapsulate them in a porous membrane (like a plastic), which would have large enough pores to let insulin out but would be too small to let the body's immune system in to attack. This microencapsulation technique is already being tried on humans. For instance, in May 1993 Dr. Patrick Soon-Shiong, of St. Vincent Medical Center in Los Angeles, injected 680,000 adult insulin-producing islet cells into the abdomen of a thirty-eight-year-old man who has had diabetes for more than thirty years. Dr. Soon-Shiong has permission from the FDA to perform nineteen more implants.

Given that this technique or some variation of it works, where are all the beta cells needed going to come from? Probably from beef or pig pancreases, just as insulin itself originally did before human insulin was created using DNA technology. Another possibility is fish insulin; yes, fish insulin from tilapia fish. This lost idea, first envisioned seventy-one years ago, is being pursued because insulin is not produced by the pancreas in this species of fish but rather the islet cells reside in separate structures, which are easy to extract. (The Japanese and Germans used fish insulin for diabetics during World War II.) One possibility is to create fish with human insulin genes. Far out? Not in the modern world of genetic engineering!

Keep watching the papers for developments. You'll be seeing a lot of headlines like "Diabetes Cure in Sight." Unfortunately, when you read on, you'll probably discover that the "fantastic" breakthrough has been with three mice in New Jersey.

In time, however, we're confident that a real cure will be here. What you have to do in the meantime is keep your spirits up, keep your diabetes under control, and keep yourself in the best possible shape so that you'll be able to, as Mary Ellen Baran put it, "Hop onto your own star when it comes your way."

Will diabetes shorten my life?

In the past the statistics about the shortened life expectancy of diabetics have been, to say the least, depressing. The old estimate of life expectancy for diabetics was that, *all things being equal,* diabetes shortens a person's life by one-third. But that estimate is now questionable because of the advent of blood-sugar testing and the immense increase in the number of people who are in good control. But for the sake of argument, let's accept it. What, then, does "all things being equal" mean?

Our interpretation is that if you do *not* have diabetes and yet you live the way diabetics do—you eat a perfectly balanced diet low in fats and sugar; you drink little or no alcohol; you do not smoke; you keep your weight slightly below normal; you get regular daily exercise and regular nightly sleep—you will live one-third longer than a diabetic doing the same thing.

But let's face it. Without the incentive of a chronic health problem to make them follow such an optimum life-style, ninety-nine people out of one hundred won't do it. No, better make that 999,999 out of 1 million.

Now, let's say all things *aren't* equal. You don't have diabetes. You are overeating—and eating all the wrong things—overdrinking, oversmoking, and carousing around and never exercising, except possibly in occasional violent weekend spurts. Will all this shorten your life? Yes, very likely more than diabetes will.

We can't offer any guarantees, but as Dr. Oscar Crofford of Vanderbilt University pointed out at the 1980 American Diabetes Association annual meeting, we already know that poorest control of diabetes is associated with highest risk of complications, while near-perfect control is associated with the lowest risk. So if you follow the recommended diabetic life-style, keep your blood sugar in good control, and keep your risks down, it is our unshakable belief that you can bring your span of years up to and even beyond that of the average person who is either unaware of the principles of good health or disinterested in following them.

A concrete testimonial to our theory is that over 1,102 people have been awarded the Fifty Year Duration of Diabetes medal by the Joslin Diabetes Foundation in Boston. The medal is given to people who have successfully lived fifty years or longer as insulin-dependent diabetics. This is a considerable achievement, because many people who earned the medal got diabetes before insulin was available. This means their early years with diabetes were particularly dangerous and detrimental. These people are the true heroes and heroines of diabetes. And there would be many, many more medal winners except that the Joslin Foundation requires complete medical records. There are also a large number of potential winners who haven't bothered to apply for the medal.

Naturally, if you ignore your diabetes and the good health principles it requires you to follow, you can make all the depressing statistics come true. So the real question is, Will *I* shorten my life? And only you can answer that one by the way you follow the diabetic program of diet and exercise.

How can I avoid the complications of diabetes?

We have mixed emotions about ranting at you about diabetes complications. Some doctors and nurses feel that unless they paint vivid horror pictures, diabetics won't take their disease seriously and do what they should to take care of it.

Sometimes this backfires, though, as we learned in a letter from one diabetic. On the first day of her diagnosis and hospitalization, she was told by the head nurse, "You have a dreadful, dreadful, dreadful disease." The nurse convinced her that all she had to look forward to was "becoming a blind, bilateral amputee, carried off to dialysis three times a week." This experience so affected her psychologically, she wrote, that

> I lay awake night after night shaken with an unbearable fear. It permeated every aspect of my daily life. I gave up wearing contact lenses because I cried so much. I was worn out emotionally. My college doctor suggested psychiatric counseling. I was hesitant, but after six months I was helped greatly and started taking better care of myself because I finally felt there was a glimmer of hope for the future.

On the other hand, we can't just ignore or gloss over the complications. They can happen, but you have it in your power to make them *not* happen by keeping your diabetes under control—that is to say, keeping your blood sugar normal most of the time.

Many people involved with diabetes, either as patients or health professionals, have long believed that it's possible to avoid complications by keeping blood sugar in or near the normal range. As diabetic diabetologist Richard K. Bernstein, M.D., stated years ago, "Diabetes doesn't cause complications; poor therapy causes complications."

But still there has been an ongoing debate on the subject. Despite the anecdotal evidence and passionate proselytizing by those of us who were True Believers in tight control, many health professionals remained unconvinced. They were unwilling to impose a more rigorous regimen on their patients without incontrovertible scientific proof that the effort would pay off.

With that Diabetes Control and Complications Trial study we mentioned previously, the proof is here. The debate is over and, as one of the physicians presenting the results in June 1993 said, "The clouds of uncertainty have cleared. Good diabetes control significantly prevents complications." You can bet your life on it. Literally.

The DCCT was conducted at twenty-nine American and Canadian medical centers. Over a ten-year period it followed 1,441 people with Type I diabetes. The patients in the study were divided between those using the "conventional" diabetes treatment of taking only one or two shots of insulin a day and one blood-sugar test and those using a more "intensive treatment." This intensive treatment involved taking three or four shots of insulin (or using an insulin pump that continuously delivers small amounts of insulin) and doing a minimum of four blood-sugar tests a day. Even though the blood-sugar levels of those using intensive treatment were still somewhat above those of nondiabetics, they were much closer to normal than those using conventional therapy. The mean daily blood sugar of the intensive group was 155; that of the conventional group was 231.

Dr. Orville Kolterman, head of the University of California, San Diego, test site, called the conclusions of the study "fairly spectacular." And so they were. Diabetic retinopathy was reduced by 76 percent, kidney disease was prevented or delayed by 56 percent, and neuropathy (nerve damage) by 60 percent. Since the study groups were relative young (ages thirteen to thirty-nine) and in relatively good health, there were not enough cardiovascular incidents to prove that the intensive treatment would be of help in preventing those, but one of the doctors in charge said that even in that area "the trends are very encouraging."

But how about people with Type II diabetes? Does tight control help them as well? The American Diabetes Association in their Position Statement says that it's not known for certain, but they conclude that it seems reasonable to recommend tight control in many Type II patients since it is presumed that the cause of complications would be the same in both types.

The morning after the results of the study were made public, Mary Tyler Moore, who was on more of a conventional therapy for her diabetes, appeared on "Good Morning America." When asked if the study might cause her to change to a more intensive therapy, she responded, "I'm changing today!"

The interviewer asked her if she'd had any complications besides the retinopathy for which she'd received successful laser treatments. She said she didn't think so, but added, "Diabetes is like a great-looking house that has termites. You never know what's going on in there."

Good control is like tenting and fumigating that house and getting a lifetime guarantee that the termites are gone.

How do I keep my blood sugar normal?

You asked the question correctly: "How do *I* keep my blood sugar normal?" Because diabetes is the original do-it-yourself disease. Although you'll have help and guidance from the health professionals on your diabetes team, the responsibility for day-to-day therapy is all yours.

Normalizing blood sugar involves many aspects of your life and lifestyle. You need a good diet, preferably one tailored to your needs by a dietitian, a sound exercise plan that you can stick to, some stress-control techniques that appeal to you and work for you, and self-education with magazines, books, and lectures to keep your knowledge growing. That will about do it for the great majority of you. Some Type II people will need to take pills, and some will need insulin. All Type I people will need insulin.

Now we come to the key question of what normal blood sugar is. The normal range is around 60 to 140 milligrams of sugar per deciliter of blood. (Milligrams per deciliter is usually abbreviated to mg/dl.) We think the objective of most all diabetes treatment should be to keep blood sugar within this range; in other words, in tighter control than in the DCCT study. Ideally, each person's goals should be set individually. As was stated when the DCCT results were announced, "No formulas can be applied to every patient and therefore intensive therapy must be used with prudence and common sense." This caution applies especially to people with heart problems, the elderly, and those Type I's subject to sudden, severe attacks of low blood sugar. They may be advised for safety's sake to keep blood sugars in higher ranges.

After you eat, your blood sugar rises and reaches its peak between a half hour and one hour later. In nondiabetics it rarely goes over 150. Blood sugars above 160 suggest that a person is diabetic. Here is the normal pattern of blood sugar for nondiabetics in relationship to meals:

Relation to Food	Blood-Sugar Range
Fasting (before breakfast)	60–100
1 hour after meal	100–140
2 hours after meal	80–120
3 hours after meal	60–100

Diana Guthrie, a professor of nursing at the University of Kansas School of Medicine in Wichita, has provided us with this chart of recommended blood sugars for diabetics.

Relation to Food	Ideal	Acceptable
Fasting	80–110	120
1 hour after meal	100–150	180
2 hours after meal	80–130	150
3 hours after meal	80–110	130

You'll notice that on these charts the blood sugars you should aim for have both a lower boundary and an upper one. Although diabetes is primarily associated with blood sugars that are too high, insulin-taking diabetics often run the risk of having blood sugar that is too low. Low blood sugar, known as hypoglycemia, can result from too much insulin, too little food, too much exercise, etc. We will go into the details of hypoglycemia in the section for insulin-dependent diabetics. Type II diabetics who take pills can sometimes experience hypoglycemia, but it is milder and less frequent. We'll discuss that in the section for Type II diabetics.

Can anything besides eating and not eating make my blood sugar go up or down?

Yes, and you need to take these factors into account. Blood sugar often goes up when you have an infection—the flu, the common cold, stomach upsets. Major surgery and pregnancy cause a rise.

Then there are a number of drugs that tend to raise blood sugar: caffeine, oral contraceptives, estrogen, and cortisone are the most important to know about. Emotional tension also causes blood sugar to swing upward.

Besides being lowered by fasting or by insufficient food, blood sugar goes down when you exercise strenuously. Among drugs with a lowering effect are alcohol (when you don't eat while drinking), large doses of aspirin, blood-thinning drugs, barbiturates, and sulfonamides.

For a complete list of medications that increase or lower blood-sugar levels, see the Reference Section: Medications that increase or lower blood-glucose levels.

How will I know if my therapy is working?

You take tests. Most of your testing will be self-testing. In a sense, you are your own laboratory technician. Here are the tests you will learn to perform or have performed.

Blood-sugar test. Your most important and most frequent test is a blood-sugar test. Only by testing your own blood sugar can you tell from day to day how well your therapy is working. And only if you make a record of your test results can your doctor see how good your control is or what modifications in your treatment are needed to improve it.

Thanks to modern technology, self-blood-sugar testing, called "monitoring," is getting faster and more trouble-free. Your results are available in between twenty seconds and two minutes, depending on the system you're using. Blood-sugar testing is performed by putting a small drop of your blood on a pad. Then you compare the color that the pad turns to a color chart (the less expensive method) or you use an electronic meter to interpret the blood sugar from the pad and give you a digital readout. This is more expensive but more accurate. Some of the newer meters use an electronic sensor rather than a chemically treated pad.

Most diabetes health professionals consider the development of self-blood-sugar testing to be the greatest advance in diabetes treatment since the discovery of insulin in 1922. Everyone should take advantage of it.

Type I diabetics typically need before-meal and after-meal tests, before-exercise and before-driving-a-car tests, and tests whenever they feel symptoms of low blood sugar. Almost all Type II's need tests before breakfast (fasting) and some one-hour-after-meals tests. Those on medication (pills or insulin) need before-breakfast and before-supper tests plus some after-meals tests.

Granted this kind of careful self-care means using a lot of those expensive testing strips. If finances are a problem, there is one thrift measure you can take, but you'll have to settle for the less accurate visual testing. You can cut Chemstrips bG in half lengthwise, thereby getting two tests for the price of one. Plus you'll have the additional advantage of using a smaller drop of blood. (If you determine your insulin dose by your blood-sugar test, visual testing is not recommended.)

Hemoglobin A_1C test. Another test for assessment of control that all diabetics should use is the hemoglobin A_1C test, also called the glycosylated hemoglobin test. This test, combined with daily blood-sugar readings, gives you a total picture of your diabetes control, as it provides you with the long-range view.

An A_1C test should be taken about every three months. The A_1C test is a laboratory test that is taken in your doctor's office. It analyzes how much glucose (blood sugar) has bonded with your red blood cells. This measurement indicates what your average blood sugar has been over the past eight to ten weeks. The A_1C test aligns closely with risks for diabetes complications. That's why it's important to have it taken about every three months.

Urine test. Before blood-sugar testing came on the scene, urine testing was the only way we had to know how well our diabetes was being controlled on a day-to-day basis. When blood sugar goes too far above normal, usually 150 to 180, some of the sugar spills over into the urine so that the body can get rid of it. Measuring the amount of sugar in your urine was supposed to indicate your blood-sugar level, but it was very inaccurate because:

- It indicated only what your blood sugar had been, not what your blood sugar was at the time of test;

- it couldn't tell you if your blood sugar was too low (hypoglycemia);

- it could be affected by such things as the amount of water you'd been drinking and any vitamins you'd been taking; and

- not everyone spills sugar when their blood sugar is between 150 and 180. Older people often don't spill until it's much higher (June doesn't spill until she's over 220), and children can show sugar in their urine when it's lower than 150.

So our advice is to forget urine testing except when you need to test for ketones.

Ketone test. You'll remember that ketones are the substances that accumulate in the blood and subsequently in the urine when glucose can't get into the cells and you burn your own fat and muscles for fuel instead of the carbohydrates you eat, which are normally the body's fuel.

Years ago there was a fad diet that had people eating only protein and fat (no carbohydrate). They were to test their urine for ketones every day and to be happy when they found ketones in it, because it meant they were burning fat and therefore losing weight.

Diabetics should *not* be happy to find ketones in their urine. In fact, if you find them, you should contact your doctor immediately for advice on how to get rid of them because their presence means you are seriously out of control.

How do I test for ketones?

A better question might be, *When* do I test for ketones? The answer for Type I diabetics is whenever two consecutive blood-sugar tests are over 200. For Type II diabetics who still produce insulin of their own, the situation is not so crucial, but all diabetics need to watch for ketones when they have infections, illnesses, or out-of-the-ordinary emotional stress.

The brand-name products to use for urinary ketone tests are Chemstrips K and Ketostix. You can also test for ketones using Chemstrips uGK and Keto-Diastix, which measure sugar in the urine as well.

What's the most accurate blood-sugar meter?

It's the one you find easiest to use. Ninety-nine percent of meter accuracy depends on the operator. That's why all the meter manufacturers try to make their instruments as operator-independent as possible: "No buttons, no wiping, no blotting, no timing, no cleaning," etc. That's also why they come up with such self-descriptive names as "One Touch" and "Easy."

In truth, all meters function well. The FDA must approve a meter before it's released to the public. They're all tested extensively. You can find the results of the required laboratory tests somewhere in each company's operator's manual, usually under a heading like "Performance Characteristics." Here you can read all the statistical gobbledygook (correlation coefficient, standard deviation, etc.) that proves the meter to have acceptable accuracy.

This leads to a corollary on the other side of the accuracy coin. When people report that a meter is inaccurate, what most of them should be saying is, "I can't operate this meter correctly" (or, if they really do know how to operate the meter correctly, "I don't like what this meter is saying about my blood sugar, so it must be wrong"). The technical-services department of one meter company reported that 90 percent of the meters returned to the company as reading inaccurately were operating perfectly.

How do I select the meter I can operate most accurately?

The answer to this is simple: select the one your doctor or diabetes educator recommends. This is true for several reasons. It is usually the meter they use in their own office. It will therefore be easy for them to check out your meter (and your technique) any time you come into the office. Having the same meter as your health professional will give both of you confidence in the accuracy of your own test results. Health professionals have their prejudices, too. They often think the meter they have—and are most familiar with—is the only truly accurate meter.

Some doctors also have a machine that prints out your blood-sugar readings from a specific meter. In that case, they'd want you to have the meter that's compatible with their machine. Be sure you find out *exactly* which meter they recommend before you go shopping. Have them write down the name for you, because meter names are very similar and it's easy to get them confused.

If your health professional has no particular preference, you need to find the meter that's best suited to your lifestyle, economic situation, manual dexterity, visual acuity, blood volume, aesthetic taste, and whether the strips for the meter are covered by your health plan. To figure out all this, you'll need to read the brochures of all the meters or, better still, see all the meters in person and have someone knowledgeable explain the features of each. That kind of service is very rare these days, because there are now so many meters, each company spinning out a new version every year or so, that no diabetes center or supply house can make them all available or afford such a large instructional staff. For that reason you need to use almost as much care in selecting where you buy the meter as in selecting the meter itself.

Where should I get my meter?

Try to find a diabetes-supply outlet or teaching center or pharmacy that will give you personal instruction in operating the instrument. This is particularly important for those who have never taken their own blood sugar, not even with a visual strip. First-timers must learn how to get a drop of blood from a finger stick and apply it to a test strip. This maneuver requires a very special technique for each type of strip. Strips come in all sizes and forms. Some are foil-wrapped and not easy to open. Some are tricky to load into the meter. Some require much more blood than others. Some absorb blood easily while with others it wants to skate off. Even if you have to pay more for the meter, get as detailed a lesson as you can, including having your instructor watch you perform a sample test and critique your technique. Go back for a second training session if you feel insecure.

How much should I pay?

Meters run the gamut in the sophistication of their technology and in their cost. Depending on how basic or advanced the meter is, where you buy it, and whether you pay or have the outlet bill your insurance, pricing goes from free or under $50 (often with a rebate and/or trade-in) up to around $200 (with kits that provide all essential supplies).

In buying a meter, remember, the meter itself is a one-time expense; what you really need to consider most is the price of the strips that are used with it. Each year they go up, all of them in lockstep. Some are as high as 80 cents each. A new trend of advantage to consumers is the availability of reduced-costs brands manufactured by competitors of the meter companies.

Our philosophy is to buy the meter you're most happy with if you can possibly afford it. A meter you find compatible with your skills and life-style is a great bargain compared to a cheap one you'll leave on a shelf to gather dust.

The final essential consideration is the customer service and reliability of the company that manufactures the meter. The best companies offer total support: an 800 telephone number, twenty-four-hour customer service staffed by polite and knowledgeable personnel, overnight replacement of ailing meters, help and advice with operational problems. And you need a company that's large enough to have wide distribution of its strips so that you aren't locked into buying them at very few outlets. A meter with limited strip availability is a handicap and a hassle.

It's a nice dividend if the place that sells you the meter will also handle your insurance claims, but if your choice is between a place that gives good instruction and doesn't make claims and a mail-order company or pharmacy that does, you're better off choosing the instruction and making the claims yourself, unless your insurer doesn't let you.

How can I be a smart shopper?

The lowest prices on meters, strips, and all other supplies are from the mail-order companies who advertise in *Diabetes Forecast* and other magazines and newsletters. The convenience is great, too, because you don't have to drive there, park, and stand in line. But there are lots of bewares on this subject.

Since they don't give instruction, buy a meter by mail order only if you're an experienced operator who's upgrading and can learn from a manual, a tape, or a video (some companies supply free training videos). And be sure to order supplies far enough in advance so that you won't run out before the next shipment arrives.

The smart shopper doesn't just worry about price. He or she takes great pains to learn the brand names of every item used with the meter. Otherwise, on your first shopping trip to replenish supplies you'll run into a lot of trouble. You may end up with the wrong product and not be able to return it if you opened it. And the brand names of all diabetes supplies are often confusingly similar. Our advice is to take along your empty containers or write down the names of the supplies you need and take the list with you.

How can I know my meter is delivering correct results?

It's only human to worry about the accuracy of your meter—especially when it gives you a number you don't like or can't explain. After all, you're using the meter to guide you through your therapy and you want to make certain it's not sending you off in the wrong direction. But some people go too far with their suspicions. They get to the point that they spend more time and effort fiddling and fretting with their meter, taking it back for a replacement or a totally different meter, than they do actually testing their blood sugar and figuring how to improve their therapy to get better results.

Human though this "inaccurate meter syndrome" may be, you should try to avoid it. It's far better to regard your meter as a friend who wants to help you rather than an enemy out to thwart you. Here's a little self-analysis that may help you build a better and more productive relationship with your meter.

- Are your expectations of the accuracy of meters beyond their present capability? We find that people have a mistaken notion of the preciseness of meter readings. Meters give you a *range* of correctness, not one figure that represents your absolutely correct and specific blood sugar at that moment. If you get a number within 10 or 15 percent of your actual blood sugar, that's great. That's all you need to know for good control. Take that figure and adjust your food, exercise, or medication according to your doctor's guidelines.

- How is your technique? Most of the inaccuracies in meter results are due to operator error. You might want to go to your doctor or diabetes educator or the place where you purchased your meter for a review lesson and technique check.

- How clean is your meter? A dirty meter is an inaccurate meter. You should have a regular meter-cleaning schedule and also clean it anytime it looks as if it needs it. (Cleaning is not a problem with certain new meters such as the MediSense ones that use an electronic sensor that extends out from the meter so blood never touches the machine itself.)

- Do you want a way to verify that your meter is functioning properly? Use the control solution that comes with your meter—or buy new if it's out-of-date—and test your meter with that. (Hospitals do this every morning. Or at least they're supposed to!) These solutions have a preset glucose level. Some companies have them for normal, low, and high ranges. If your control test falls within the range printed on the solution insert, then your meter is AOK. Don't be surprised at the broad range considered acceptable. It may be something like 88–123 or 85–157.

- Does your test result make absolutely no sense to you? Then do a second test and see if it comes out near the first or tells you something different that you can believe. If the second test falls within the same ballpark and you're still dubious, buy some Chemstrips bG and do a visual test. A visual test is mainly good for checking if you're very high or very low, but even so it can help you settle your controversy with your meter. (Incidentally, it's not a bad idea to keep visual strips around in case your meter goes completely bonkers or kaput or you drop it and break it or take it somewhere and lose it.)

■ Are you truly upset and desperate? Call the 800 number of the meter manufacturer and see if they can help you ascertain if your reading was correct. Besides, it will give you some relief just to explain your problem to someone and maybe yell a little bit.

A final piece of advice for everyone about meter results. Whenever you go to the doctor's office and have a blood-sugar test taken there (they always want to do their own), take your meter and do a test yourself the moment after they finish. If your result comes within 10 or 15 percent of theirs, you'll go home at a good comfort level with your meter. Warning I: Don't take your blood sugar at home before you go to the doctor and expect it to be the same as the test in the doctor's office. That's how many people start developing the "inaccurate meter syndrome." The passage of time and the stress of being in a doctor's office can make dramatic differences in your blood sugar. Warning II: If there's a great discrepancy between the reading on the doctor's meter or lab test and your meter, it could be that yours is right and theirs is wrong. Stranger things have happened.

What can I do if I have trouble getting enough blood for the test?

First, try to relax. When you're tense, your blood tends to leave your extremities and go to your body organs to prepare you for the flight-or-fight response. You can tell if you are relaxed if you have warm hands.

Then make sure you're using the correct tip for your lancing device. Some of them have a choice of tips, one with a larger opening that makes a little deeper penetration than the normal tip. If you've checked that out and still have trouble, try some (or all) of the following:

1. Wash your hands with soap and very warm water. Allow warm water to run over your hands and wrists for at least one full minute. (Be sure you dry your hands thoroughly before starting your test.) Incidentally, washing your hands is much preferable to cleaning with alcohol. Not only does alcohol, when used repeatedly, dry out your skin, but if it hasn't evaporated before you take your test it can change the reading you get—usually making it lower.

2. Let your hand hang loosely by your side and shake it for at least thirty seconds.

3. Keeping your hand below heart level, milk the palm of your hand all the way up to the fingertip. Make sure the fingertip turns pink.

4. Prick the meaty side of the finger—not too close to the cuticle but not directly in the center (pad) of the finger or at the very top of the fingertip.

5. Allow your finger to relax for three to four full seconds before trying to squeeze the blood out. When you're cut or stuck with a sharp object, the muscles tighten up to prevent the release of blood. After a few seconds they relax and the blood flows easily again.

6. Milk your finger starting with the base on the palm side and working all the way up to the fingertip. Wait two or three seconds between milkings.

How do I keep a record of my blood-sugar readings?

It's great that you realize you should keep track of your blood-sugar readings. Blood-sugar testing is not an end in itself. You don't just test your blood sugar, look at the result, and say, "Nice test, there" or "Rotten test there," and go about your business. The results of your tests are important information to give health professionals so that they can analyze and evaluate them to see if your control can be improved. If you don't keep accurate records, they can't do the best job for you. The records are also valuable to you in seeing patterns in control—and lack of control.

Many blood-sugar monitors now have memories ranging from one test all the way up to 300. But even if you're using a meter with a memory, you need to write down your test results in a log book so they can be quickly viewed and assessed from the point of view of deviations from your target ranges. Most meter companies provide one log book with the initial kit, but after you fill that one you have to keep buying them (usually for around $1 each). One good log book that's free is given out by the insulin company Eli Lilly. It's called *Managing Your Diabetes Self-Care Diary.* Diabetes-supply centers and pharmacies often keep these on hand for customers.

Incidentally, if you enter all your blood-sugar tests in your log book, you can then add them up periodically and calculate your average blood sugar. Oddly enough, this correlates very well with an A_1C test. That is to say, if your average falls within the normal scope (70–140), you would probably come out in the nondiabetic range on an A_1C test also. And doing an average is a heckuva bargain compared to $40 for an A_1C lab test plus a doctor's office visit. In the *Diabetes Self-Care Method,* Drs. Peterson and Jovanovic-Peterson explain that if you take a measurement before each meal and a second one about an hour after you've eaten, the sum of the six tests should add up to about 600, and that gives you an average blood glucose of 100. Perfect!

Another excellent record booklet is *Charting: The Systematic Approach to Achieving Control,* by Janice Roth, R.N., C.D.E. This contains detailed daily records for food, exercise, stress, etc., and a simpler monthly calendar. The daily recording system shows you how to analyze your body's responses and create a personalized program for control. (*Diabetes Self-Management,* Book Division, 150 West 22nd Street, New York, NY 10011; price is $5.45 including shipping.)

How can I learn more about taking care of my diabetes?

Read books. Read periodicals like *Diabetes Forecast, Diabetes in the News, Diabetes Self-Management, Diabetes Interview,* and *Diabetic Reader* (see Recommended Reading).

Join your local affiliate of the American Diabetes Association (see Reference Section: Directory of Organizations) and attend their meetings. They usually have guest speakers—podiatrists, dietitians, ophthalmologists, or other professionals—who can fill you in on their own areas of expertise and answer questions that may have been puzzling you. Diabetes associations often sponsor day-long seminars with different speakers, panel discussions, and workshops. These are a terrific way to get a lot of diabetes information in a short period of time.

Find a diabetes education program in your area. Ask the ADA for names and places or write to the American Association of Diabetes Educators (see Reference Section: Directory of Organizations). These education programs sometimes charge a nominal fee, but you always get a lot more than your money's worth.

Diabetes education programs can involve a one-week crash course or weekly meetings over a period of time. They can be inpatient programs for newly diagnosed diabetics in the hospital, but most are outpatient. They can involve large or small groups, or they can offer individual instruction. There may be a group of teachers (nurses, dietitians, psychologists, social workers, etc.) or there may be one diabetes educator who handles the whole course. As you can see, you can usually find a program to meet your needs, whatever those needs may be.

Another way to learn is from other people with diabetes by sharing helpful information, experiences, and mutual concerns. There are over 800 diabetes support groups in the United States. Our favorite psychologist, Dr. Richard Rubin, tells us of the benefits of such a group. "The good ones help people feel less isolated, more comfortable with their diabetes, and more able to do the right thing when it comes to their self-care. In addition, support groups are free or, at most, require a small contribution. That's a real benefit, I encourage people to join support groups. Look for one you like and keep looking until you find one."

Ask your doctor and your diabetes educator and call the closest ADA and JDF offices to find a group. If you can't find one, start one yourself. And how do you do that? You ask someone who has done it successfully, like Bettie Norgord, founding mother of the Dynamic Sharpshooters, a group that in ten years has grown to 340 members.

For advice and counsel, contact Bettie Norgord, 4677 W. Earhart
Way, Chandler AZ 85226 (Phone: 602-940-9377).

Where can I find out about the latest developments in diabetes therapy as soon as they happen?

You could read diabetes publications. But a surer method is to keep
track of the *business* of diabetes. Business magazines and
newspapers like *The Wall Street Journal* often beat *JAMA* and
the *New England Journal of Medicine* in announcing new diabetes products. Better still, ask a stockbroker to send you prospec-
tuses of companies involved in diabetes research, equipment, and
products.

For example, we have a stockbroker friend who recently sent us
information on Amylin Pharmaceuticals, Inc. Their initial entry
into the diabetes market, now almost at the end of its Phase II trials,
is Normylin, an analog of a natural peptide hormone produced, like
insulin, by the islet cells in the pancreas. Insulin and this hormone
regulate the body's glucose metabolism. Normylin (AC 137), used
as a replacement hormone along with daily insulin injections, is
purported to help Type I's, who lack the hormone, avoid hypoglycemic attacks. This could be an advantage for people using the tight
control therapy of the DCCT, because the major drawback of that
therapy is the increased risk of hypoglycemia.

This company is also developing a product—AC 253—for
Type II people. It seems that Type II's sometimes have an excess of
that natural peptide hormone just as they often do of insulin and this
excess may be responsible for their insulin resistance. AC 253 is designed to restrain the effect of the hormone and prevent the resistance.

The company predicts that these new products will be on the
market by 1998. With this two-pronged attack, they're expecting to
do great things for diabetes—and for themselves: an anticipated
$830 million in sales the first few years! Thereby hangs the tale of
how developments in diabetes equipment and products generally

come about. Not to discount altruism, but considering the growing diabetic population, it's not surprising that many companies are entering the field with big-time profits in mind. But whyever the developments occur, we'll be happy just so long as they do occur and make diabetes therapy easier and better.

Cautionary note: our friend said that most new drugs or technologies don't work even though they seem promising at the outset. So when you read about spectacular new products that sound like just what you need, don't let your hopes—or your investment dollars—get out of hand.

DIABETES AND YOUR EMOTIONS

How can I keep from being depressed over my diabetes?

It's not easy. It's only logical to be depressed when you first learn you have diabetes. And all the cheerful remarks people make about how much nicer it is to have diabetes than leprosy or than being run over by a moving van or some such nonsense do no good at all. You know that it's *not* better than having nothing wrong with you.

After all, you have to make many, many changes in your life, and at first glance these changes all seem to be for the bad. On top of that, you feel like an outcast. You're no longer like everyone else. Of course, no one ever *is* like everyone else, but at the moment you feel like the town pariah, and you're certain that all your friends are going to drop you now that you have diabetes.

You get the automatic "why me?" reaction. "Why should *I* be selected to get this rotten disease?" "Why should *I* be threatened with blindness or kidney failure or gangrene or an early death if I don't follow a rigid regimen?" Why indeed? There's really no reason. It's just the breaks of the genetic game. As a doctor told us once at a meeting, "Every person carries around about forty-four genetic defects." One of yours happens to be diabetes, and the fact is that some people draw out far worse tickets than diabetes in the genetic lottery. But that doesn't make you feel any better. As A. E. Housman said, "Little is the luck I've had/and, oh, 'tis comfort small,/to think that many another lad/has had no luck at all."

So what do you do about all this? You can sit and resentfully mutter about cruel fate and wallow in your woe, or you can, as the old saying has it, take the lemon you were handed and make lemonade out of it. We read an article about a woman who is a successful author and consumer advocate on radio and TV in Los Angeles. She described her beginnings: "When we married, during the early years it was rough. We were poor, but I wasn't about to go on welfare. So I decided if I wanted clothes, I had to make them. If I wanted the best bread I'd better learn how to bake. What I did was take poverty and turn it into an art."

What you need to do is take diabetes and turn it into an art. Do all the things you need to do for your diabetes and make them enhancements to your life.

How do I turn diabetes into an art?

The beginning step is to accept the fact that you have diabetes. The first thing most people do with diabetes is to deny it. Oh, your mind may know you have diabetes, but everything else about you—your heart, innards, soul, imagination, all those things you really listen to—say, "This has nothing to do with me. I'll ignore it and it will go away."

Alas, it won't, and you'll never be able to practice the art of diabetes until you get rid of the idea you don't have it. As a matter of fact, you need to do more than just accept your diabetes. One young woman, after hearing us speak at a diabetes meeting, said to June, "You actually seem to embrace diabetes." That she does. Not that she wouldn't prefer not to have diabetes, but since she does have it, she's determined to squeeze all the good out of it she can.

What's good about having diabetes?

Without being ridiculously Pollyannaish about it, we can affirm that diabetes *does* do some positive things for you. This isn't just our idea. Many diabetics have written to us and told us about what they consider to be the advantages of diabetes.

For one thing, you learn the principles of good health. Until you're whammed with something dramatic like diabetes, you may just bumble along wrecking your health through bad habits, laziness, and ignorance. Diabetes teaches you the right way to live and gives you a reason for doing so. As one diabetic skier put it, "This disease, this condition will keep you healthy and fit for whatever your heart desires."

Diabetics often actually feel better than they did before having their disease. Young diabetics have reported to us that they do better in sports than their nondiabetic friends because they never eat junk food and always keep regular hours. They're in top-notch shape all the time. Professional motorcycle racer Michael Hunter says unequivocally, "If I didn't have diabetes, I wouldn't be as good as I am." Well-controlled diabetics also say they're less susceptible to colds and flus that their friends pick up with seasonal regularity.

Diabetics often look better than their nondiabetic contemporaries. Conscientious diabetics are lean and vital, bright of eye and quick of step. People of the same age who don't have diabetes to goad them onto the path of healthful living are often pudgy, sallow, and lethargic.

Diabetes develops self-discipline. Young persons who have diabetes and must assume responsibility for their own care develop a mature attitude of self-sufficiency at an early age. The discipline of following the diabetic way of life carries over to school and work and sports and creative endeavors. It can help make you a successful person in all areas of living.

Sometimes diabetes even sparks ambition. We know a young diabetic woman who is a successful city attorney. She told us how her choice of a profession came about: "When I got diabetes in high school I knew I'd have it all the rest of my life. I realized it would be an expensive disease, and I decided I wanted to always be able to take care of myself—and take care of myself *well*—whether I ever got married or not. That's why I worked hard to prepare myself for a good career."

And having diabetes makes you more compassionate toward

others with problems. You learn how to give help gracefully and receive help without embarrassment or resentment. This, after all, is what puts the humanity in human beings.

But perhaps best of all, diabetes makes you capable of change. To change is the hardest thing for people to do. That's why so many of us take the easy way out and stick in a rut for our entire lives, unable to rouse ourselves into action to make the changes that could make us into the persons we were meant to be.

Diabetes, because it requires changes, and rather dramatic changes at that, shows you that you *can* change. If you can change in one area, then you are capable of change in other areas. You can improve not only your health but your whole life.

How do I start making all the changes I have to for my diabetes?

You phrased that correctly. *You* have to make the changes. As psychologist Dr. Richard R. Rubin said in *Psyching Out Diabetes,* "No one can make anyone else do anything." Try as they may, health professionals and concerned family members and friends can't force you to make the changes your diabetes requires. And they certainly can't do it for you. It's all up to you.

As we said before, your first step is to wholeheartedly acknowledge that you have diabetes and that it's here to stay. That gets you halfway to change land. The next step is to—as the new psych jargon puts it—*empower* yourself: realize that you *can* control your diabetes and your health and your life. Now you're three-quarters there. All that's left for you is to make those changes.

At this critical point we often hear the plaint, "I just can't get myself motivated to _____ (exercise, test my blood sugar, lose weight, change my diet, etc.)." What will get you over the motivation hurdle into change? Dr. Rubin says it can be something positive like falling in love, wanting to have a baby, or becoming a grandparent. Or it can be something negative like the first harbingers of a complication. But you're buying high-priced trouble if you wait around until fate brings you a wonderful positive motivator or you

start feeling the first twinges of neuropathy. It is far better to motivate yourself as did a young woman from Hawaii who wrote to us.

*Motivation is the reason I'm writing. Your book deals with the
diabetic who can't seem to get motivated. I've also heard this from
diabetics I've met in Hawaii who are still feeling sorry for themselves rather than doing something. My motivation is quite simple. I
look down at my two feet and thank God they are attached to two
legs. I also thank God that my eyes function so I can see those feet. I
want to keep my feet and keep my eyes. THAT is motivation. As much
as I love food, there is no food tempting enough for me to give up my
feet or my eyes. So whenever temptation comes along, I just look
down at my feet.*

Those feet can make that important final step into change.

But so much of the change seems to be giving up pleasures. How can I feel good about that?

We found that when June, in her early fits of depression, was ticking
off all the pleasures she'd have to give up because of diabetes, what
she was really ticking off were habits. Something like eating a sweet
dessert was a habit that she considered a pleasure merely because
she'd done it so often that it was a comforting part of her daily routine. The trick is to establish new *good* habits and turn them by constant use into pleasures.

This is not as hard as you may think. Eating a delectable, juicy
piece of fresh fruit can become as much of a habit-pleasure as eating a big, gloppy dessert. For many people a daily bike ride or after-
dinner walk is a pleasurable habit, and it can become one for
you, too.

Furthermore, when you're thinking of the things you have to
give up because of diabetes, think of these: you have to give up ever
waking up with a hangover, either of the cigarette or alcohol variety;
you have to give up discovering on a shopping trip that you've bal-
looned another dress or suit size; and you have to give up feeling and
looking like a couch potato because of lack of exercise.

Finally, if, as you make the changes in your life, you still have moments of depression, try to keep in mind that it's part of the human condition to be depressed from time to time. There will be a natural tendency for you to lay your every woe on the doorstep of your diabetcs. That's unfair to diabetes. Bad though it may be, it's not enough of a villain to be responsible for every dismal moment in your life. Even if you didn't have diabetes, you wouldn't be frisking around in a constant state of ecstasy. Though they call life the human comedy, it isn't all laughs for anybody.

But it isn't all tears, either, and you should make every effort to emphasize the good aspects of your life—to make yourself into a happy person.

How do I make myself happy?

You just do it. As Mark Twain said, "Everyone is just about as happy as he makes up his mind to be." And Robert Louis Stevenson believed that "there is no duty we so much underrate as the duty of being happy." So make up your mind and do your duty. It's vital that you do so for an important reason.

Not that you need a reason to justify happiness. It's a perfectly wonderful end in itself. But the reason we have in mind has only recently come to light. Studies reported in the *New York Times* show that being a happy, good-natured person can make you healthier, and that being an angry, suspicious person can be literally lethal: "People who are chronically hostile, who see the world through a lens of suspicion and cynicism, are particularly vulnerable to heart disease."

But that's not all. According to Dr. Ray H. Rosenman, a cardiologist at the SRI International Research Institute, hostile people are more prone to die prematurely from *all* causes, including cancer. They even get minor ailments like colds and the flu more often than happier people.

Your anger doesn't have to be the explosive, blow-your-top variety, either; more subtle styles of hostility—skepticism, mistrust, a tendency to make snide comments—are just as damaging. Strangely enough, even competitive, hard-driving type-A personalities who are not hostile are less at risk than their more antagonistic counterparts.

Try this experiment. The next time you feel hostile and angry, take your blood sugar. Assuming your negative feelings aren't due to low blood sugar, you'll probably discover your blood sugar ascending. Conversely, when you feel happy, take it and you may find, as June did once when she was looking forward to a trip to San Francisco, "I'm so happy I can't keep my blood sugar up."

Another reason to try to cut back on your anger is because of what it does to those around you. Many diabetics are angry because they have diabetes, but they don't like to admit the source of their anger, not even to themselves, so they displace their anger onto something or someone else. It could be the doctor's bill or the meter that gives a high blood-sugar reading or the health professional who's trying to help them make changes in their lives that they don't want to make or even their loving family members and friends.

The worst thing about displaced anger is that if you never admit its true source, you'll never get rid of it. It will keep festering within and erupting without.

Even if you acknowledge that your anger is diabetes-related, how do you deal with it? Dr. Richard Rubin explains that anger is "a signal that something is wrong, that you're feeling vulnerable, scared, hurt, embarrassed, attacked or overwhelmed. This causes you to react in one of three ways: (1) passively by burying your feelings, (2) aggressively by lashing out with anger, or (3) assertively by dealing straightforwardly with the situation." Dr. Rubin's book *Psyching Out Diabetes* shows how to handle anger assertively, as well as how to rid yourself of other negative emotions like depression, fear, and frustration that cloud your existence and block out the sunshine of your life. If you can't find this book in your library or bookstore, write to Prana Publications, 5623 Matilija Ave., Van Nuys, CA 91401, or call 1-800-735-7726.

How does getting emotionally upset affect my diabetes?

An emotional upset has about the same effect on blood sugar as chocolate-chip cookies. A fight with an intimate, a boost in rent, a week of final examinations—any stressful event in your life can send diabetes dramatically out of control. The strange thing is that even if something favorable takes place in your life, that, too, can sometimes raise your blood sugar. When we were consultants on a tour to Hawaii for diabetics, several of the participants told us they got out of control with the excitement of packing for the trip.

Our own experience has convinced us that if you're working very hard at good control and usually achieve it but find that during certain periods there is a change for the worse and you can't figure out why, try getting out from under your normal life situation, especially if it's more hectic than usual. You may find, as June frequently does, that there's nothing wrong with your diabetes therapy, but that there *is* something wrong with your life and that *that's* what needs to be changed.

We are so convinced of the need for diabetics to learn how to handle the stresses of contemporary life that we wrote an entire book on the theme. The revised edition of *The Diabetic's Total Health Book* explains why tensions and stresses have a negative effect on diabetes, what stressors you can avoid, and how to develop techniques to keep those you can't avoid from upsetting your control. A good portion of that book is devoted to instruction in relaxation therapies. These therapies—exercise, self-hypnosis, biofeedback, meditation, and guided imagery—are the best preventive medicine ever invented. Each of you should start practicing the ones that appeal to you most. You'll particularly enjoy practicing our unique all-purpose relaxers: laughter, travel, pets, and hugs, all of which will enhance your life and the lives of all those around you. *The Diabetic's Total Health Book* is also available from Prana Publications.

DIABETES AND YOUR DIET

What is the diabetic diet?

You hear a lot of talk about "the diabetic diet," and we ourselves sometimes fall into the trap of using that term. In reality, though, there is no one diabetic diet.

In the first place, the general diabetic diet is not a diet in the way most people think of one—a rigid and unnatural eating pattern that you follow until you remove extra pounds, at which time you revert to your old way of eating (and almost invariably put the pounds back on again). It's more a lifelong eating plan that should do three things for you:

Keep your diabetes under control. Your diet is of primary importance in controlling your blood sugar. For good control, Type I diabetics should focus on counting carbohydrates, since carbohydrates are primarily what is converted into glucose, which raises your blood sugar. Type II's should concentrate on lowering the amount of fat in their diet and adding fiber in order to level out their blood sugars.

Keep you healthy. Important as it is to keep your diabetes under control, that's not enough. You're much more than just a case of diabetes. You're a whole living person, not just a pancreas, and you need to eat a healthy diet for that whole living person. We're always amused to see those exchange lists for fast-food establishments that make it look as if you could follow the exchanges, eat fast food for every meal, and live healthily ever after. You can't. You need to follow the general principles of dietary health, just as everyone else interested in longevity and feeling good does.

Let you enjoy your meals. Julia Child, the famous French-style gourmet cook, who's very frisky at the age of eighty, complains that Americans are becoming afraid of food and they're eating it as if it were medicine, when they should be thinking of it as healthful and tasty and a pleasurable social experience. She's right. Vive la Julia!

The American Diabetes Association and the American Dietetic Association now recommend that diabetics eat, on a per meal basis, a diet of 55 to 60 percent carbohydrate, 12 to 20 percent protein, and 20 to 30 percent fat. (All foods are composed of various combinations of carbohydrate, protein, and fat.) These are the same proportions of nutrients that are recommended as health enhancing for all Americans. Most of us are still overeating both protein and fat. Some people's diets are as high as 40 percent fat, and most of that fat is the worst kind—saturated or animal fat, which causes high cholesterol. For diabetics, a particular worry is that it can make insulin less effective.

The American Diabetes Association's booklet *Exchange Lists for Meal Planning* (available from the ADA for $1.30 plus $1.75 for shipping) is designed to help you, working with your dietitian or doctor, plan a daily diet so that each of your meals has approximately the same number of calories and the correct amount of carbohydrate, protein, and fat. The ADA exchange lists group together foods that are alike. There are six food-category lists from which you choose: starch/bread, meat and meat substitutes, vegetables, fruits, milk and milk products, and fats. You are assigned a certain number of choices (exchanges) from each list for each meal. So it becomes easy to plan meals of great variety but similar nutritional content.

The lists also indicate which food choices are high in sodium, fat, or fiber. Sodium and fat should be limited. Fiber should be increased, because it helps slow down the effects of foods that might otherwise send blood sugar soaring. There is a special *Exchange Lists for Weight Management* for people needing to lose weight. In addition, there are three supplements for special dietary problems: *Guidelines for Use of the Exchange Lists for Lowfat Meal Planning, Guidelines for Use of the Exchange Lists for Low-Sodium Meal Planning,* and a combination of the two, *Guidelines for Use of the Exchange Lists for Low-Sodium, Lowfat Meal Planning.*

An alternative diet especially beneficial for Type II diabetics is the one created by Dr. James Anderson of the Veterans Administration hospital in Lexington, Kentucky. Dr. Anderson was the original champion of oat bran in this country. His plan, the High Carbohydrate Fiber (HCF) nutrition plan, is helpful for overweight non-insulin-dependent diabetics. It can lower insulin requirements and eliminate the need for pills in many Type II diabetics. (For books explaining this diet, see Recommended Reading.)

Just the opposite diet is recommended by Dr. Richard K. Bernstein of Mamaroneck, New York. His book *Diabetes Type II; Including New Approaches to the Treatment of Type I Diabetes*

emphasizes absolute normalization of blood sugar by severely restricting carbohydrates to 6 grams at breakfast, 12 grams at lunch,
and 12 grams at dinner. His is per force a high-protein-and fat diet.
He believes that "loading with carbohydrate will probably be more
harmful in the long run than loading with fat."

Dr. Lois Jovanovic-Peterson, who coauthored *The Diabetic
Woman* with us, thinks that dietary recommendations should always
be based on a person's type of diabetes. In her opinion, the ideal
diet for one type of diabetes may worsen control in another type.
She points out that the goal of diet is to help maintain normal blood
sugar, so the ideal diet for each person is the one that facilitates
keeping that person's blood sugar normal. Thus diets must be individualized. Only your blood-sugar tests can tell you if your diet is
working.

For all these reasons and because there are so many dietary options, we think working with a dietitian is the best way to find the
eating plan that is right for you.

How can I find a dietitian?

If there isn't one on your doctor's staff, ask for a recommendation or
call the local hospital and ask for a recommendation.

You might also get in touch with the local affiliate or chapter of
the American Diabetes Association, or write to the American Dietetic Association for a list of names of dietitians in your area. You
could also contact the American Association of Diabetes Educators. Many members of this organization are dietitians with a particular interest and expertise in diabetes. (See Reference Section:
Directory of Organizations.)

Sometimes dietitians are listed in the yellow pages of the telephone directory. They may be listed under "Nutritionists" as well.
But you have to be careful. There are some strange types who call
themselves nutritionists and may try to put you on seaweed and soybeans and promise you the moon (that is to say, a cure). Stay away
from these at all costs (and their costs are likely to be high; the moon
is an expensive commodity).

Make sure the dietitian is an R.D.—a registered dietitian. And try to find one who has enough imagination and knowledge to open up meal possibilities geared to your own tastes and needs and not one who just gives the same food prescription to all diabetics.

How do I find out how many calories a day I should be consuming?

Again, the best way is to consult your dietitian, who will assign you the correct number of calories to eat. Sometimes your doctor is the one who does this for you. The Joslin Clinic in Boston has a neat formula by which you can work out the number of calories you need if you know what your weight should be (see Recommended Reading). Relatively inactive people should eat eleven calories per pound of body weight a day. Active people need around fourteen calories per pound. To lose weight, the clinic recommends eating less than eleven calories per pound a day—ideally, about nine. To gain weight, eat more than eleven calories per pound each day, say between fourteen and sixteen.

Also, you have to remember that men can eat more calories than women and that growing children and adolescents use more energy and need more food than adults or older people. We once read a rule of thumb that after the age of forty, people need about 10 percent fewer calories each decade if they want to stay the same weight. That's exactly the kind of information we all hate to hear, but it does have validity in nutritional circles.

Table 1 on page 45 can be used as a general guideline.

How can I make myself follow the diabetes diet?

You can conjure up horror stories in your imagination about the terrible things that will happen to you if you don't. But a strong, positive approach is better. Make your meals so delicious and interesting that you *want* to follow your diet. Make your eating not a grim therapy, but a pleasurable delight. There are lots of gourmet cookbooks available for diabetics (see Recommended Reading). Try new recipes. Try variations on old recipes. Try different herbs and spices

TABLE 1.
Calorie Allowance for Adults for Various Body Weights and Ages, Assuming Light Physical Activity

Median Body Weight of Men		Daily Calorie Allowances According to Age		
lb	*kg*	*22*	*45*	*65*
110	50	2200	2000	1850
121	55	2350	2150	1950
132	60	2500	2300	2100
143	65	2650	2400	2200
154	70	2800	2600	2400
165	75	2950	2700	2500
176	80	3050	2800	2600
187	85	3200	2950	2700
198	90	3350	3100	2800
209	95	3500	3200	2900
220	100	3700	3400	3100

Median Body Weight of Women		Daily Calorie Allowances According to Age		
lb	*kg*	*22*	*45*	*65*
88	40	1550	1450	1300
99	45	1700	1550	1450
110	50	1800	1650	1500
121	55	1950	1800	1650
128	58	2000	1850	1700
132	60	2050	1900	1700
143	65	2200	2000	1850
154	70	2300	2100	1950

Data from Food and Nutrition Board, National Academy of Sciences, National Research Council: Recommended dietary allowances, ed. 8, Washington, D.C., 1974, U.S. Government Printing Office, p. 29.

(most of these are free, diabetically speaking). And don't overlook the aesthetics of food serving. A few flowers on the table give you no extra carbohydrates or calories and do a lot toward making mealtimes a pleasure.

This all holds especially true if you live alone. June, in her prediabetic days, often used to have for dinner what we called an "avocado sandwich maybe," since whenever someone asked her what she was having for dinner, she usually responded vaguely, "Oh, I guess I'll have an avocado sandwich maybe." Which meant she had no idea what she was going to have and didn't intend to make any plans. She was going to grab whatever she found in the refrigerator, if anything.

Now June always has a well-planned and delicious meal that she eagerly looks forward to. Her appetite is also better. And strangely enough, although she's eating fewer calories, she's eating more—and more satisfying—food. This is because she's cut down on high-calorie fats and entirely cut out high- (and empty-) calorie junk foods.

The most ghastly diabetic diet idea we've ever heard of is the result of a man's decision that calculating the diabetic diet is too much of a chore. He resolved to eat the same breakfast, the same lunch, and the same dinner every day. Ugh! Besides being lethally boring, this is nutritionally unsound. Diabetics need a lot of variety in their diets in order to make certain they're covering all the nutritional waterfronts. Not only that, but, as a home economist told us wryly, "you should eat a great variety of foods because there are so many chemicals in everything these days, it's the only way you can avoid getting a big buildup of one chemical that might cause harmful side effects."

Which foods are best for keeping my blood sugar normal?

First, you have to realize that it is mainly the carbohydrates in foods that are converted directly into glucose and affect your blood sugar. True, about 65 percent of protein becomes glucose, but since it takes six or eight hours to do so, it has more of a stabilizing than an escalating effect. Fat is not changed to glucose—one of its few virtues for diabetics.

But all carbohydrates are not created equal. There was no scientific data on what effect individual carbohydrate foods have on blood sugar until 1983, when Dr. David Jenkins and fellow researchers at the University of Toronto published the Carbohydrate Glycemic Index (see Table 2). This is a classification of how high and how fast certain foods raise blood sugar. The problem with the index is that in compiling it only sixty-two foods were tested.

For diabetics, generally speaking, a food with a low (slow-releasing) glycemic index is preferred to one with a high (fast-releasing) index. The foods on the index are compared to glucose, which is assigned the top figure of 100. The findings are often surprising: sucrose (table sugar) is only 59, while carrots (cooked) are 92; instant potatoes are 80, but sweet potatoes are only 48. Ice cream is only 36, so index-wise it's as good for diabetics as lima beans, which are also 36. If you're thinking there must be a catch, there is. A bowl of ice cream has a lot more calories—and the wrong kind—than a bowl of lima beans. In other words, you cannot and should not eat by glycemic index alone. Blood sugar is not the only factor to consider; calories and nutritional values count, too.

It's also known that when carbohydrates are eaten as part of a meal that includes protein and fat rather than alone, blood sugar rises less. A further complication is that not all people respond to different kinds of carbohydrate in the same way. In a sense, you need to use your blood-sugar tests to figure out how you respond to different food. You need to create your own glycemic index.

Though there are these drawbacks to the glycemic index, we find that it is for many people a very helpful guide to foods likely to help or hinder control. Eating more of the foods with an index of 50 or lower and less of those with higher ratings might make an encouraging difference to many of you who have been innocently consuming too many foods at the top of the scale.

Do I have to measure my food?
Yes. It's the only way to be sure you're getting the amount of food your diet specifies, neither more nor less. *Exchange Lists for Meal*

TABLE 2.
Carbohydrate Glycemic Index

Simple Sugars
Fructose—20   Honey—87
Sucrose—59   Glucose—100

Fruits
Apples—39   Bananas—62
Oranges—40   Raisins—64
Orange Juice—46

Starchy Vegetables
Sweet Potatoes—48   Instant Potatoes—80
Yams—51   Carrots—92
Beets—64   Parsnips—97
White Potatoes—70

Dairy Products
Skim Milk—32   Ice Cream—36
Whole Milk—34   Yogurt—36

Legumes
Soybeans—15   Garbanzos—36
Lentils—29   Lima Beans—36
Kidney Beans—29   Baked Beans—40
Black-eyed Peas—33   Frozen Peas—51

Pasta, Corn, Rice, Bread
Whole-wheat Pasta—42   White Bread—69
White Pasta—50   Whole-wheat Bread—72
Sweet Corn—59   White Rice—72
Brown Rice—66

Breakfast Cereals
Oatmeal—49   Shredded Wheat—67
All-Bran—51   Cornflakes—80
Swiss Muesli—66

Miscellaneous
Peanuts—13   Sponge Cake—46
Sausages—28   Potato Chips—51
Fish Sticks—38   Mars Bars—68
Tomato Soup—38

Planning gives portions in cups and tablespoons or teaspoons as well as in weight. Unfortunately, this sometimes leads to sizable variations in amounts, so you should stick to ounces and actually weighing. Type I people, especially, need to be careful to eat portions of the correct size in carbohydrates. This is where a food scale comes in handy.

Using bagels as an example, our science-trained friend Daisy Kuhn, a professor of microbiology, gave us a great lesson in carbohydrate variation in the starch/bread exchanges on the lists. Each serving on the starch/bread list is supposed to have about 15 grams of carbohydrate and eighty calories. For a bagel exchange, the list says "½ (1 oz.)" as the amount to eat. In actuality, not many half bagels are only one ounce (approximately 30 grams). To check on this figure, Daisy bought some bagels at a local deli. Using her Soehnle food scale, she found that a half bagel weighed 2¼ ounces, and therefore contained 33⅘ grams of carbohydrate. As a Type I diabetic she knew that if she hadn't weighed her bagel she would have eaten over twice the carbohydrate she wanted to and probably would have run up a high blood sugar. Type II's, of course, would be eating twice the calories they wanted to, as well as possibly too much carbohydrate.

Likewise, a slice of bread should be limited to one ounce. But what a difference there is in reality between most supermarket bread and what you find in health-food stores or in bakeries. So get yourself a Soehnle or equivalent scale and do some weighing, at least at the beginning of your new eating plan. We ourselves still weigh bread and also pasta before we cook it. The *ADA Exchange Lists* also suggests, "A scale can be very useful to measure almost anything, especially meat, poultry and fish." It points out that most meats weigh less after cooking and that many starches (pasta, rice, oatmeal, lentils, etc.) become much larger in bulk when cooked. Or, even better, use the easy way to weigh food and convert it to exchanges—buy a Diabetic Exchange Center food scale. Manufactured by Health-O-Meter, a division of Continental Scale Corporation, it gives you the weight of your food in ounces and then converts this to food exchanges. It is available at the many diabetes-supply centers and at some diet centers.

If you're really conscientious at first about weighing and measuring your food, you'll be amazed at how quickly you learn to eye-measure or, as with bread, hand-weigh when you're out to dinner at a friend's house or in a restaurant. (Hint: sometimes it helps to discreetly nudge your food into little piles, the better to estimate the quantity.) You may get so good at eye-measuring and hand-weighing that you can do weight- and quantity-guessing parlor tricks, like the guy who guesses weights at the circus. Of course, the real and worthwhile trick is using your skill to eat the exact amount of food on your diet.

Can I skip some breakfast and lunch food exchanges and save them for a big dinner?

That's not a good idea for people with diabetes, especially when that big meal is at night. Your metabolism is slower at night and caloric needs lower than at any time during the day. Smaller, more frequent meals and snacks are the preferred way of life.

You'll get into real trouble by trying to follow the great American eating pattern of nothing much for breakfast, a light lunch, and a gorging session at night. According to the book *Outsmarting the Female Fat Cell,* by Debra Waterhouse, M.P.H., R.D., typical Americans eat 70 percent of their calories after five o'clock at night, whereas Europeans and other cultures eat their largest meal at midday. Her theory is that that's why these cultures do not have the weight problems that Americans do.

Studies have actually shown that Type I's who skip meals and eat one large meal at night have poor glucose tolerance, higher cholesterol levels, and, again, a tendency to be overweight. Type II's run the same risks plus an even greater tendency for weight gain.

Is there anything I can eat all I want of without counting it in my diet?

You can hype up the flavors of your meals with herbs and spices without counting them. And you can eat as much of the following vegetables as you want, if you eat them raw: chicory; Chinese cabbage; endive; escarole; iceberg, butter, red-leaf, or romaine lettuce; parsley; and watercress. There is a list of such "free foods" in *Exchange Lists for Meal Planning.* You can also eat all the unsweetened rhubarb, unsweetened cranberries, and unflavored gelatin that you can possibly hold. Yum!

Can I follow a vegetarian diet?

Of course. We consider the vegetarian diet extremely healthy for everyone and especially good for non-insulin-dependent diabetics who are overweight. In fact, Dr. James Anderson's HCF diet (see reference to this diet on page 42) is as close as it can get to a vegetarian diet without being one.

One advantage of vegetarianism is that the diet is naturally low in fat and high in fiber. Many of the staples of the diet—soybeans, beans, oats, lentils, pasta, rice—are low on the Carbohydrate Glycemic Index (see page 48). This, along with their high fiber content, means that food becomes glucose at a slow pace and blood sugar stays normal more easily. In addition to helping control diabetes, a vegetarian diet reduces the risk of heart disease and tends to promote weight loss.

There is more than one type of vegetarian diet; *vegan,* or no animal food at all; *lacto-vegetarian,* all vegetable except for milk, cheese, and other dairy products; and *lacto-ovo-vegetarian,* in which both dairy products and eggs can be eaten. The problem with vegan is that calcium and iron may be in low supply and a pill supplement may be advisable. The main problem with all vegetarian diets is that they can be deficient in vitamin B-12, which can be taken in pill form but is more effective when injected. So if you're an insulin taker and familiar with the injection process, you might ask your doctor about shooting your own B-12.

To follow a vegetarian diet as a diabetic, you need special food lists for guidance in calorie content and carbohydrate and fat amounts. The most complete lists we know of are in Marion Franz's *Exchanges for All Occasions.* Our favorite vegetarian cookbook is

The New Laurel's Kitchen, which, unlike many such cookbooks, is not laden with sweets and fats. See Recommended Reading for a complete list of exchange lists and cookbooks.

Will I be able to follow my diet in restaurants?

Of course. It won't be as easy as following it at home, where you can select and measure everything to make sure you're getting exactly what you need, but with a little experience and ingenuity it can be done. In fact, it is done by diabetics every day.

At first, when you're just getting started with diabetes, you might want to check out the restaurant ahead of time to see what they have on the menu that would be right for you. This gives you time to figure out in advance what you want to order. You can also find out if they have, for example, fruit for dessert rather than something gloppy and sweet. If they don't, you can bring along a piece of fruit and either eat it there or eat it after you leave.

Checking out the restaurant ahead of time is also a good idea because you'll know if it's open. Sometimes on a trip June has gone out to a restaurant recommended in a travel book or article only to find it's been closed for six months. This can be more than an awkward situation if it's time to eat and there's no other restaurant around.

For insulin-dependent diabetics, a reservation is very important. The person taking the reservations should be informed that one of the diners is a diabetic, that the table *must* be ready at the time of the reservation, and that the food *must* be served without undue delay. (None of this sitting around in the bar for an hour waiting for a table, which happens in a lot of restaurants that may be trying to get you to buy extra drinks.)

What kinds of things should I order in restaurants?

As long as you avoid concentrated sweets, you can usually order anything you want. At first, though, try to avoid unfamiliar concoctions that are likely to have a lot of sauce (sauces often contain a great deal of carbohydrate and fat). Straightforward poultry or fish, and bread and vegetables are the easiest things to recognize and measure.

This doesn't mean you're stuck with plain fare. A recent book, *The Restaurant Companion,* by Hope S. Warshaw, R.D., C.D.E., takes the mystery out of ordering meals in fourteen kinds of restaurants. It includes ordering models and exchanges for eight ethnic cuisines, including Mexican, Chinese, Italian, Thai, and gives advice for salad bars, brunches, and airline meals—all potentially dangerous situations. You may want to take this book to the restaurant with you and consult it as needed. (Try your local bookstore or call Prana Publications.)

What do you mean by concentrated sweets?

Concentrated sweets are what, when you taste them, are sweet, all sweet, and nothing but sweet. They're sugar, honey, and syrup. They're candy, frosted cake, pies, cookies, and ice-cream sundaes. They're almost everything listed on restaurant menus as desserts. They're all soft drinks, except artificially sweetened ones.

Concentrated sweets are an assault upon your system that sends your blood sugar soaring. Besides that, they quickly use up your daily allotment of calories without giving you any real food value in return—empty calories, as they're known.

Are there any sweeteners I can safely use?

Sweets are a problem for all of us. We seem to be biologically programmed to like them. Our ancestors had to have this craving for sweets to inspire them to climb trees for fruit to get the vitamins they needed. Or it may be psychological, because we were rewarded with sweet treats when we were good little girls and boys, and we still seek that feeling of being loved and approved. Or it may be a combination of the two, and that makes it even harder to kick the sweet habit.

Let's talk first about the ubiquitous sugar (sucrose) before we take up the rest. You've probably been terrorized about even so much as looking at a grain of it. But now we're being told that a little bit of sugar is no problem in a well-balanced diet. Scientists have concluded that it does not cause a more rapid rise in blood-glucose levels than starch. Just don't eat more than 10 percent of your total carbohydrate calories in the form of sugar (they're empty calories) and never use it straight in drinks. As our Type II book collaborator, Virginia Valentine, says, "You can have goodies such as low-sugar cookies (animal crackers, gingersnaps, vanilla wafers, etc.), low-sugar cakes with no icing, or low-sugar frozen yoghurt or ice cream."

There are two kinds of sweeteners: noncaloric and caloric. The noncaloric sweeteners include saccharine, aspartame (NutraSweet and Equal), cyclamates, and Sunette (Sweet One). The most commonly used caloric ones besides sugar are fructose, sorbitol, mannitol, and HSH. Caloric sweeteners should not be "ingested freely," as dietitians like to put it. We actually don't feel that *any* sweetener should be ingested freely, since you never know when a laboratory mouse is going to clutch his bladder or liver and topple over and cause hysterical headlines about a previously approved sweetener. So again you have that good old boring admonition to practice moderation.

One way of achieving moderation is not to concentrate on one kind of sweetener but to vary them, never having more than a couple of items sweetened with any one kind of artificial sweetener a day. That way if the mouse topples, you won't have to worry that your system is loaded with lethals.

Following is a rundown of the various sweeteners and how to fit them into your diet.

Caloric Sweeteners

Fructose. There are several good things to say about fructose. First off, it's not an artificial sweetener. It is, as they like to say about almost every product you see in markets these days, "all natural." It is found in sweet fruit and most vegetables. It is also available in granular and liquid form in diabetes supply centers. It tastes sweet and has about the same calorie count as sugar (one hundred calories per ounce). But because it is much sweeter than sugar, you can use less of it to get the same sweet taste. The graph on page 56, reprinted from *Laurel's Kitchen,* shows how much sweeter it is.

Fructose also doesn't raise your blood sugar as fast or as high as sucrose. The Carbohydrate Glycemic Index (see p. 48) gives it a 20 as compared with a 59 for sucrose and a 100 for glucose. One caution: *if your blood sugar is already high, fructose will raise your blood sugar just as fast and as high as sugar.*

If you want to use fructose in baking, our former dietitian Ron Brown suggests that you use it for one-quarter of the sugar in the recipe and a noncaloric sweetener for another quarter. You can usually just leave out the rest, he says, since most desserts are too sweet anyway.

The British Diabetic Association reports that when you use fructose in cakes, it tends to keep them fresher longer and also has a better taste than ordinary sugar. The association does caution, however, in capital letters and boldface type: **FRUIT SUGAR IS NOT SUITABLE FOR THE OVERWEIGHT.**

There have been reports that fructose raises triglycerides (fats stored in the blood). However, at the 1993 ADA Scientific Sessions this fear was put to rest by John P. Bantle, M.D., with the statement that fructose has no effect on triglycerides. But it does raise cholesterol, primarily the LDL's (bad ones). This is now the main objection to fructose in the diabetic diet. Once again, moderation is the answer in using any kind of sweetener.

The terms *fructose* and *fruit sugar* are used interchangeably. In England and Europe, fructose is usually made from fruit; in the United States, it is made from corn. Fructose and fruit sugar are chemically the same, although some people claim there is a difference in taste.

Sorbitol. Sorbitol, a sugar alcohol found in many plants, like fructose, doesn't cause the blood sugar to rise as rapidly as sugar because of the way it's metabolized. Sorbitol suffers a bad press for its tendency to have a laxative effect in certain susceptible people. (We think of that as nature's way of promoting moderation.) We've also

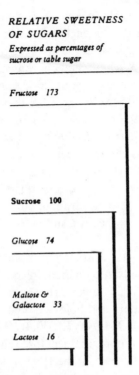

RELATIVE SWEETNESS
OF SUGARS
*Expressed as percentages of
sucrose or table sugar*

Fructose   173

Sucrose   100

Glucose   74

Maltose &
Galactose   33

Lactose   16

Reprinted by permission from *Laurel's Kitchen* by Laurel Robertson, Carol Flinders, and Bronwen Godfrey (Nilgiri Press, 1976).

heard people denigrate sorbitol as an artificial sweetener. Not true. Sorbitol is found naturally in fruit. It was our friend Daisy Kuhn, professor of microbiology at California State University at Northridge, who put us straight on this. She even gave June a basket of prunes and pears as a sorbitol Easter gift, explaining that these two fruits are among the highest in sorbitol. This, of course, explains why prunes work so well as a laxative. Other fruits with a high sorbitol content are plums, berries, apples, and cherries. Daisy tells us that it is safe for most adults to eat about 40 grams of sorbitol if it is spaced out over a day. A three-ounce serving of prunes has about 12 grams of sorbitol. Hard candies sweetened with sorbitol contain about 2.6 grams. Though many commercial foods are sweetened with sorbitol, consumers in the United States cannot buy it for home use.

Another erroneous bum rap for sorbitol is that it causes the diabetes complications of retinopathy and neuropathy. This is a confusion between two different sorbitols. The sorbitol that does the damage is a waste product produced from glucose in the bloodstream. It is definitely *not* the sorbitol eaten as food. (Incidentally, an enzyme called aldose reductase stimulates the conversion of blood glucose into sorbitol. For that reason a new drug is being developed to block the action of aldose reductase and thereby to prevent the development of these diabetes complications.) To reiterate: *sorbitol eaten as a food is not implicated in eye, nerve, or kidney damage.*

Mannitol. Mannitol, another sugar alcohol, is similar to sorbitol—including its laxitivity in susceptible individuals. It's also used as a commercial sweetening agent, although not as commonly as sorbitol.

HSH (Hydrogenated Starch Hydrolysate). Daisy Kuhn tells us that HSH is *chemically* the same as sorbitol. We've heard that it isn't quite as laxative as sorbitol, but since we've heard this mainly from companies that manufacture products made with HSH, we're waiting for more evidence to substantiate this claim. HSH is the sweetener in many sugar-free candies.

Noncaloric Sweeteners

People have very strong feelings about artificial sweeteners. Some won't touch them with a twelve-foot tongue. One woman called us in a fury to cancel her subscription to our newsletter because we mentioned Equal in it. And we once heard a lecture by a doctor, a medical adviser for an ADA chapter, in which he cited the many evils of saccharine, saying that it, and not cyclamates, should have been banned by the Food and Drug Administration. (He's been at least half vindicated, since the FDA has for several years been reviewing a petition for its reapproval; it may soon be back on the market in the U.S.) By the way, any of the artificial sweeteners tasted alone will taste anywhere from bad to funny. They taste good only in foods and drinks. Here, then, is a brief rundown of the current crop of artificial sweeteners.

Saccharine. This is the primary sweetening component of Sweet 'N Low and Sugar Twin. It can be used in cooking. Some people find that it has a bitter or metallic aftertaste, but when combined with fructose in a recipe it's not noticeable. Because saccharine has been known to cause cancer when fed to animals in huge amounts, the FDA requires all products containing saccharine to bear the following warning: "Use of this product may be hazardous to your health. This product contains saccharine, which has been determined to cause cancer in laboratory animals." Those studies haven't yet been directly correlated to humans.

Aspartame (NutraSweet and Equal). This is currently the most popular noncaloric sweetener around—and it is around everywhere. It doesn't have the aftertaste of saccharine, but its tragic flaw is that it loses its sweetness in cooking or baking and doesn't have enough bulk for baked goods. One packet of Equal is equivalent in sweetness to two teaspoons of sugar. One tablet equals one teaspoon of sugar.

Since aspartame can be harmful to people with a rare metabolic abnormality called PKU (phenylketonuria), the FDA requires that it carry a warning on the package. The FDA considers that an acceptable amount of aspartame is up to fifty milligrams per kilogram (2.2 pounds) of body weight. Gloria Loring, in her *Kids, Food, and Diabetes,* translates this as one twelve-ounce can of aspartame-sweetened soda per 12 pounds of body weight. Actually, a 132-pound person would have to consume eighty-six packets a day to reach the FDA's maximum accepted intake.

Cyclamates. Until cyclamates are back on the market, we won't know the equivalences of the packages. We do know that a lot of people will be welcoming cyclamates back, especially those who've been doing their cyclamate runs to Canada during the years it has been banned in this country. People like the fact that it has no aftertaste and that you can cook with it.

Keep watching the newspaper for announcements of its return and the inevitable warning and praising articles that will appear in its wake. It is not yet known what kind of FDA warning it will have to bear—if any.

Sunette (Sweet One). Sunette was safely used outside the United States for five years before it was approved here. It's the only dietetic sweetener that doesn't require a warning label. (Apparently so far nary a mouse has toppled.) Sunette is two hundred times sweeter than sugar. Its big advantage is that it doesn't break down when heated; therefore, you can cook with it. Each packet gives the sweetness of two teaspoons of sugar, and each contains four calories and one gram of carbohydrate. The carbohydrate is in the form of dextrose. "Not to worry," says our dietitian Meg Gaekle. "It's added only to give bulk." (The manufacturers of Sweet 'N Low do the same thing.) In the small amounts generally used, it causes no problems.

A final reminder: honey, molasses, pure maple syrup, and other such sweeteners are not approved for diabetics no matter how many ill-informed health-food-store people tell you they are. For more information on sweeteners, see the Reference Section: How Sweet It Is.

What do I do if I am served too much food?

Leave what you can't eat or, in the case of expensive protein, take it home with you in a doggie bag. (You may have enough meat to last you for two or three meals.) June has the trick of carrying plastic bags in her purse and quietly bagging any excess.

One way to avoid getting plates that are bursting with calories is to go to restaurants that feature California or spa cuisine. But don't be sad if there aren't any of these in your area. They are usually very expensive, and you can actually sometimes get too little food in such establishments.

A happy trend in restaurant menus is the appearance of special "Pritikin Plates" and American Heart Association selections. These are low in calories and fat and high in fiber; watch for them. You should also watch for the restaurants that have special "light eater" dinners. There aren't many of these, but there are more and more all the time, because more and more people want to watch their weight or, as in the case of older people, just have diminished appetites.

Another way to get a smaller portion if you're dining with a cooperative person is to order one entree and split it. Each of you can then have an individual choice of appetizer. This limits both the amount of food and its price.

Our favorite trick for getting smaller portions and saving money and yet experiencing the best of dining out is to go for lunch rather than dinner. The portions are about half as large, with prices to match. A further advantage is that you're eating your main meal in the middle of the day, so you can walk it off afterward rather than just going to bed on a full stomach and letting it turn to fat. We especially do this main-meal-at-lunch trick when we travel. Dinner is then something light in the hotel coffee shop, or something we bring into the room.

Are salads always a safe bet when you're confused about what to order?

Let's take the ubiquitous salad bar, for example. It can be hazardous to your health in several ways. People sometimes cough and sneeze over salad bars, and to keep the ingredients fresh-looking, they are often sprayed with allergy-causing sulfides. But worst of all, while you think you're restricting yourself to a diet meal, you're actually loading up on calories from the dressing. One study showed that the average person takes in more calories from a salad bar than he or she would from a standard meat-and-potatoes lunch.

It's not always that much better if the salad is brought to your table. As *Better Homes and Gardens* reported, a chef's salad with cheese, ham, turkey, and half an egg dolloped with blue-cheese dressing has seven hundred calories and fifty-eight grams of fat. For less than half the calories and 10 percent of the fat you can have a turkey sandwich made with two slices of whole-wheat bread, lettuce, and tomato.

Since dressing is the major culprit in a salad's assault on your diet, the only way to order salad is with dressing on the side. Then don't dump big globs onto your salad, but use this little trick a dieter once taught us: dip your fork into the salad dressing and then pick up the lettuce or other vegetable with the fork. Just enough dressing clings to the fork and is transported to the salad to give it flavor with minimal calories.

Can I eat in fast-food chains?

Yes, and you can eat from the pushcart of a Tijuana taco vendor, but neither would be the best choice for your overall health. As we mentioned previously, you can follow the diabetic exchange system and presumably keep your diabetes under control in fast-food chains, but the food there is far too high in fat (especially saturated fat—the wrong kind) and sodium and far too low in fiber. But we realize there is often no other choice for a quick and economical place to eat, and we also realize that for some high-school and college students fast food is a way of life. So when you must (or choose to) eat fast food, the following books are invaluable in helping you select what in horse-racing circles they call the best of a poor field:

Fast Food Facts, by Marian Franz, published by DCI Publishing, gives the calories, carbohydrate, protein, fat, sodium, and diabetes exchanges for the food served at twenty-six chains, including Arby's, Burger King, Chick-Fil-A, Church's Fried Chicken, Dairy Queen, Domino's Pizza, Jack in the Box, Kentucky Fried Chicken, Long John Silver's, McDonald's, Pizza Hut, Roy Rogers, Wendy's, Whataburger, and White Castle. There is a good introduction on the philosophy of dining in fast-food restaurants and the pitfalls to avoid. In the analysis of each restaurant's foods, there is a forthright list of foods not recommended.

The *Completely Revised and Updated Fast-Food Guide,* published by Workman and written by Michael Jacobson, Executive Director of the Center for Science in the Public Interest, is a real feast of information. It tells what's good, what's bad, and how to tell the difference. The nutritional charts for foods at nineteen top chains include saturated fat, sugar, sodium, and vitamins, besides the usual nutrients. There is even a guide to the best choices in each chain. This book is a real eye-opener for anyone addicted to fast foods.

Another book, *The Diabetic's Brand Name Food Exchange Handbook,* published by Running Press, gives the calories, exchanges, and sodium content of 4,000 supermarket products and the same information on foods served at nine different chains. But since this book doesn't include the fat and cholesterol content, it leaves you in the dark about two of the most significant health facts.

Being informed about the actual content of fast foods—along with the amount of fiber, which none of these books documents—is what should keep you out of most fast-food chains except on rare occasions.

The latest trend in fast food is to make it somewhat healthier (*really* healthier is not possible). McDonald's has led the pack with its McLean Deluxe (91 percent fat free and 280 calories) and other chains are falling into line. They're also adding more chicken choices, but the majority of calories in these comes from fat, and beware of the sauces. Tread carefully in pizza places; choose the low-calorie vegetable toppings and remember the importance of portion size. When it comes to Mexican food have tacos or tostadas (skip the sour cream and guacamole) or even a bowl of chili.

And, finally, some chains display posters with nutritional information to help you make good decisions. Look for these at McDonald's and Burger King and elsewhere. That's a trend of genuine benefit for the wise diabetic diner.

How can I stay on my diet when I'm invited out to dinner?

First, make sure that anyone who invites you to dinner knows you're a diabetic. That shouldn't be difficult, because people who know you well enough to extend the invitation will probably have long since been informed about your diabetes.

Almost anyone who knows you're a diabetic will ask what's special about your diet. An easy way to explain it is to show the person the answer to the question "How do I plan a meal for my diabetic friend?" (see the section "For Family and Friends"). If you don't have this book handy, just be sure to mention the piece of fruit for dessert. You might add that any vegetable is fine, except those high on the glycemic index, such as cooked carrots, parsnips, and beets.

Another strategy was suggested by the Reverend Gerald Eaton, of Nicholasville, Kentucky. When he travels to other churches to preach, he sends an explanatory dietary sheet ahead to the host church. This is for those who will be providing him with meals. See the Reference Section for a copy of his sheet. He just tells them he's on a "special diet" and not that he has diabetes, because if they have a diabetic "Aunt Susie" who doesn't watch her diet, he doesn't want them to think he can eat her way.

How do I make it through the holidays without breaking my diet?

Remember the origin of holiday festivals? They were the few occasions in the year when peasants who ran around most of the time with hollow, rumbling stomachs could really fill up. Now, however, most of the people in this country aren't perpetually hungry. On the contrary, what a biologist friend of ours calls "hyperalimentation," or eating too much, is a national epidemic. The American public's overeating habits are bad enough the whole year round, but then along come the holidays with the atavistic excuse for overindulgence, and the scene becomes a dietary disaster area.

Revelers sometimes rationalize their holiday behavior by quoting the philosopher who said, "What you eat and drink between Thanksgiving and New Year's isn't all that important. What really counts is what you eat and drink between New Year's and Thanksgiving." Of course, this philosopher didn't have diabetes. Diabetes doesn't take a holiday, and a diabetic can't take a holiday from health. So what are you to do?

Now, although there are gatherings where you won't be tempted by alcohol over the holidays (for the problem of avoiding alcohol, see "Can I drink alcohol?" on page 68), there's almost nowhere you can go where you won't be tempted by food, especially sugary food. With visions of sugarplums dancing in everyone's heads and on everyone's tables, it's going to take all your ingenuity to stick to your diet or, as we prefer to think of it, your healthful eating plan.

Let's take the last first—dessert. It's not uncommon to find two kinds of pie plus fruitcake, cookies, ice cream, whipped cream, and candy being offered with nary a morsel of plain fruit in sight.

But wait. There may be *some* in sight. Look at the centerpiece. It's often a lovely display of autumnal harvest fruit and nuts. Eat it. While others give in to their addiction to concentrated sweets, just sit there and nibble upon items you've plucked from the centerpiece or other household decorations. You should rhetorically ask the host or hostess, "You don't mind if I just have a bit of this, do you? It looks so delicious I can't resist, and it's right on my diet." What can they say? It may give them a little understanding of what the diabetic diet is for future reference. You also may start a trend at the table. When others see you've had the courage to munch on the decor, they're likely to follow suit. Many people don't feel like a heavy, sweet dessert after a large holiday meal, but they don't know how to refuse. Show them how. (One warning: make sure the fruit isn't artificial before you sink your teeth in.)

If devouring the decor is beyond your powers of brazenness, or even if it isn't, a more gracious alternative is to bring your host or hostess a fruit-and-nut gift basket. You can call it a "diabetic dessert basket" and hope you'll be offered a chance to partake of it at the end of the meal.

Another way to avoid the dessert problem and yet still make the host or hostess happy is to take *one spoonful.* After all, if you've tasted the concoction, you can praise it, and that's the most important thing. It's also a way to make yourself feel less deprived.

Let's face the final reality, though. No matter how careful you are at a big holiday dinner, you're still likely to eat more than usual. But there is one survival tactic. Exercise more than usual. Do as much of the cooking and serving as you can arrange to. If you're going to someone else's house, tell the host or hostess in advance that you'd like to help pass things, clear the table, do anything that involves motion. Most people don't realize the physical effort that goes into serving a dinner. A few Thanksgivings ago June virtually singlehandedly put on a family holiday dinner, and although she ate a good bit more than her normal diet, that night she had the worst low-blood-sugar incident of her life.

After dinner is over keep the exercises going if you can. Organize a bird- or star-viewing walk, a caroling session, a tree-trimming activity, charades with lots of physical motion—anything to keep the calories burning and the blood sugar normal. The nicest part about all these activities is that they're enjoyable in themselves.

By the way, an after-dinner activity suggested by a former president of the American Diabetes Association, Dr. Donald Bell, is testing the whole family's blood sugar. Since everyone will have had an abnormally heavy meal, it will be an appropriate time to see how their bodies handled it. Because there are those genetic factors to diabetes, you may catch a relative in the beginning stages, and he or she can get an early start on controlling it before any damage has been done. It may sound a little bizarre, but it's a good idea.

What happens if I break my diet?

If you do it once, you'll probably do it again and again and again. And each time you do it and run your blood sugar up, you risk damage to the body and the development of the serious complications of diabetes—heart disease and stroke, blindness, kidney and nerve damage, and gangrene of the feet.

The classic rationalizations are "Once won't hurt," "I can get away with it," "It's Christmas," "I can't offend the hostess," "It's my birthday," and "I'll be conspicuous if I don't." Consider yourself in a worse predicament than an alcoholic. He or she has to be a total abstainer from alcohol. You have to be a semi-abstainer from food, half on and half off the wagon at all times. A very precarious perch.

There are, however, three exceptions when we think it is okay to go ahead and break your diet. In fact, we heartily recommend it. These exceptions are: (1) the day you win a gold medal at the Olympics, (2) your inaugural banquet when you're elected President of the United States, and (3) your one-hundredth-birthday party.

Of course, after all this preaching we admit that accidents will happen. Sometimes, for example, you'll inadvertently eat something that will be loaded with sugar. When you find yourself registering a high blood sugar after such an accident, there's no need for self-flagellation and heavy mourning. Occasional *accidental* lapses won't destroy you. (In fact, torturing yourself with frets and recriminations may do more damage to you than the dietary lapse.)

And, finally, to prove that we aren't as hard-line as we usually

seem, we offer for your consideration the Hog Wild variation (see
For Family and Friends: "If my diabetic child goes to a birthday
party or trick-or-treating on Halloween, is it all right to break the
diet just this once?" on page 172). But at the same time, we want to
warn you that wild hogs can easily get out of hand and break down
all barriers of self-control, and to assure you that June does not
practice the hog-wild variation. *Ever.*

Is it all right to drink sugar-free and diet sodas?

These drinks are a great breakthrough for diabetics since they allow
you to be part of the group without breaking your diet. As with all
things, though, a bit of moderation is in order. We heard of one man
who was downing over twenty cans of sugar-free soda a day. He
must have sloshed when he walked, to say nothing of the excess
chemicals that must have been assailing his system.

When it comes to sugar-free drinks, a bit of caution is also in
order. True story: Once when June was skiing in Deer Valley, Utah,
she felt very thirsty at the end of the day. The thing she wanted most
was to try a glass of the locally brewed beer, Wasatch Gold. But
she'd neglected to bring her testing things along to the slopes and felt
she couldn't risk the carbohydrates. Therefore, like the conscientious diabetic that she is, June marched over to the soft-drink dispenser, filled a carton with sugar-free cola, and drank it all down.

When she got back to the lodge she tested her blood sugar. It
was 220! She couldn't figure it out. She'd been exercising heavily all
day and had eaten and drunk only the right things. Why the high
blood sugar? Our conclusion was that it had to be the cola. The person who had filled the dispenser must have used the wrong cola mix,
either mistakenly or because they were out of the sugar-free variety.

We thought this was an isolated occurrence until we were talking with the former president of the American Association of Diabetes Educators, Kansas City diabetologist William Quick. He said
that he and some patients and colleagues had conducted an experiment in fast-food chains in Kansas City and in Harrisburg, Pennsyl-
vania. They tested the allegedly sugar-free drinks and discovered
that one-third of them actually contained sugar.

You can test your own sugar-free drinks by carrying Tes-Tape or Diastix (for checking sugar in the urine) and dip the strip or stick in the glass of soda and see how it registers.

As far as we know, soft drinks in cans are safe since their quality control is a little tighter than in mix-it-yourself establishments.

You also have to train family members and friends to watch what they're buying—and pouring. After twenty years of unmitigated alertness in sugar-free drink dispensing, Barbara absentmindedly bought a bottle of Schweppes tonic water that wasn't. For two evenings June drank it, wondering why her blood sugar was suddenly out of control every night. ("Am I coming down with something?") When she discovered the error, she was relieved to find that her diabetes hadn't become unpredictable. She was irritated with Barbara for her faulty purchase—but more irritated with herself for not taking the responsibility to always look for herself.

And a final warning on sugar-free sodas for Type I diabetics: just when you get everyone thoroughly trained to give you sugar-free drinks and nothing but sugar-free drinks, you'll probably have an insulin reaction and ask for someone to bring you a Coke *quick* and they'll dutifully grab a sugar-free one, which will do about as much good for raising your blood sugar as a cup of air. (That's another reason for always using glucose tablets for hypoglycemia: they don't make sugar-free glucose tablets.)

Why am I supposed to read the label on all food products I buy? Aren't all brands more or less alike?

Brands are not only *not* alike, they are very different. Only by reading the fine print on the label can you know, for instance, whether a certain can of grapefruit juice contains sugar. Some brands do and some don't, and it's important for you to choose a brand that is unsweetened.

It's amazing how many food products have sugar thrown in. Fruits in heavy syrup are typical. You have to really search to find the few fruits, frozen or canned, that are unsweetened. Cans of vegetables often contain sugar, as do canned meats, bottled salad dressings, frozen dinners, and endless other convenience foods. Even *salt* contains sugar—read the label if you doubt us.

There's also a confusion about many diet products. You have to realize that the term *artificially sweetened* does not necessarily mean without sugar. Drinks sweetened with saccharine often contain some sugar to counteract saccharine's bitter taste. On low-cal foods, watch for the words *sugarless* and *sugar free*. But even that's not a guarantee of safety. By law only sucrose counts as sugar, so you'll have to watch for the many chemical terms used to specify different kinds of sugars: glucose, fructose, dextrose, sucrose maltose, lactose, dextrin, and sorbitol—just to name a few (see Reference Section: How Sweet It Is, for a complete list).

One helpful innovation is that beginning in May 1994 with the new mandatory federal nutrition labels required on all packaged foods, sweeteners must all be bunched together and listed first in the ingredient list after the word "sweeteners." (Learn to read those new labels and avoid shopping mishaps.)

Incidentally, ingredient lists on labels are arranged according to the weight of each ingredient in descending order. The heaviest is listed first; the lightest, last. The lightest ingredients are usually those unintelligible chemical additives for which American food processors have become famous.

Can I drink alcohol?

Here you have one of the great diabetes controversies. Many doctors say absolutely no to alcohol. Not a drop. Others say it's all right in moderation. June has a joke that has a grain of truth in it. Question: "What did you do when your doctor said you couldn't drink?" Answer: "I changed doctors."

Actually, an excellent case can be made for a diabetic not to drink at all. Even alcoholic beverages that don't contain carbohydrate, such as gin, vodka, bourbon, scotch, and dry wines, do contain calories. If you have a weight problem, the additional calories of the drink will augment this problem. If you say, "Okay, I'll figure the calories of the drink in my diet and cut out something else," you will lose the food value of that something else you cut out and your body will be deprived of the nutrition it needs.

Then, too, drinking can get you in deep trouble, especially if you're on insulin. Alcohol lowers blood sugar unless you eat while you're drinking. If you start staggering or become unconscious on the way back to your car after a visit to a bar, the police will smell the alcohol and think you're simply drunk. This is not a scenario with a happy ending.

There is the additional possibility that the alcohol may throw off your medication or alter the effect of your insulin. Some oral drugs combined with alcohol can cause nausea, sweating, and dizziness. And an out-of-control diabetic shouldn't drink a drop.

Heavy drinking can result in long-range problems for a diabetic. The journal *Diabetes Care* reported a study by David McCullogh and others of over five hundred diabetic men. The heavy drinkers in the group had a much higher incidence of painful diabetic neuropathy than the others did.

The case *for* drinking is weaker than the one against it. For many people a glass of wine is a pleasurable adjunct to a meal. It is, in fact, for some national groups as much a part of the meal as the food. There is also the "French paradox" that people who drink two or three glasses a day of red wine (or white, according to a Kaiser Permanente Medical Center study) have a lower risk of coronary heart disease. Researchers do point out that wine drinkers may have other traits, such as a more healthy diet, that protect them. (But remember, *heavy* drinking *causes* heart disease.)

Even with your doctor's approval, however, before having a glass of anything you should do a little self-analysis of your drinking habits. We have a philosophy about diabetic drinking that we think holds true. There are two situations where a diabetic should *not* drink: The first is if alcohol means nothing to you, and the second is if alcohol means everything to you.

Whatever you drink has to be figured into your meal plan and the calories counted. Alcoholic drinks are usually calculated as fat exchanges, although you can also substitute them for bread exchanges. Naturally, you can't mix liquor with orange juice or tomato juice without counting those exchanges also. And you have to avoid such mixers as ginger ale, tonic, and other sweetened soft drinks.

The alcoholic drinks that don't contain sugar or carbohydrates are dry white wines (including champagne), dry red and rosé wines, white vermouth, whiskey, gin, vodka, scotch, rum, brandy, and tequila. A four-ounce glass of wine is about 80 calories; a four-ounce glass of vermouth is about 140 calories. The hard liquors are calculated according to their proof. The higher the proof, the more calories. As an example, eighty-six-proof alcohol is 71 calories an ounce; one hundred-proof alcohol is 83 calories an ounce. Beer is 156 calories per twelve-ounce bottle, but it also contains about the same amount of carbohydrates as a bread exchange (thirteen grams). Light beer is only 90 calories on the average and contains the equivalent of one-half bread exchange in carbohydrate. Liqueurs and cordials have to be avoided entirely as they contain sugar—sometimes as much as 50 percent sugar. Appetizer and dessert wines, like sweet sherry, port, and muscatel, are also too sweet for diabetics.

The general recommendation is to limit alcoholic beverages to 6 percent of your daily caloric allotment. For instance, if you're on a 1,500-calorie-a-day diet, you could have one four-ounce glass of wine (80 calories) or one generous ounce of eighty-six-proof liquor (71 calories) in soda or a sugar-free mixer. You could also have it in orange juice, if you counted that as one of your fruit exchanges. If you are on a 3,000-calorie-a-day diet, you could drink twice that much (but you wouldn't *have* to, of course).

Another solution is to limit your drinking to the nonalcoholic wines and beers now available. Ariél Vineyards of California produces award-winning alcohol-free wines that have less than half the calories of wines with alcohol. Zuri of Germany has a nonalcoholic Rhine wine that contains only 130 calories per bottle. Many alcohol-free beers are now on the market in different parts of the country.

Is caffeine bad for diabetics?

By reputation, caffeine has deleterious effects on your health. It has been accused of raising blood pressure, increasing blood fats, making the heart beat faster, causing nervousness and insomnia, perhaps increasing the chance for ulcers and breast cysts, and—especially troublesome for diabetics—raising blood sugar. But shucks, a diabetic has to give up so many things, and here you have a cup of coffee (or tea) that has no calories or carbohydrates or fats and is therefore "free" in the diabetic sense of the word, a drink that Melvin Konner, M.D., writing in the *New York Times,* described as a relatively safe mood elevator. Do you have to give that up, too? Maybe not.

Recent studies indicate that for most people (even those with heart conditions) caffeine causes no problem if you restrict your intake to three cups of coffee a day or less. June, who adores coffee, quickly figured out that if you drank coffee that was half decaf and half regular you could have six cups, so she started blending her own and is having enough satisfaction and oral gratification that she's not feeling the least bit deprived. If you are caffeine-sensitive or a pregnant woman or a child or have medical problems that contraindicate the use of caffeine, a better policy is to get your satisfaction from decaf drinks. Caffeine is found in many places and forms. To help you keep track of your intake, here are a few figures:

Source	Milligrams of Caffeine
Coffee (6 oz.)	110–150
Espresso, Cappuccino	60
Tea (6 oz.)	20–46
Diet Coke (12 oz.)	45.6
Diet Pepsi (12 oz.)	45.6
Hot cocoa (6 oz.)	2–8
Sweet dark chocolate (1 oz.)	5–35
No-Doz (1 tablet)	100
Excedrin (1 tablet)	65

What about health foods for diabetes?

If you mean home-baked bread, yogurt, soybeans, sunflower seeds, wheat germ, alfalfa sprouts, and all that, great! The more different foods you eat, the better. Just make certain that you know the calorie, protein, fat, and carbohydrate content (or exchange equivalent) of whatever you eat and limit your portions so that you stay within your diet.

June adores many health foods but finds she has to select them carefully, because many of these foods are laced with concentrated sweets—honey, coconut, dried fruits, brown sugar—and many of them are overpotent in fat and calories. For instance, one-half cup of sunflower seeds contains 280 calories and twenty-six grams of fat.

Most health breads are also heavier than ordinary bread. One slice will often equal almost two starch/bread exchanges instead of one. You can check this out by weighing a slice. Bread is usually 50 percent carbohydrate, so a slice weighing sixty grams contains thirty grams of carbohydrate, or two starch/bread exchanges.

DIABETES AND YOUR HEALTH

What should I expect from my doctor?

Maybe we should start off with a modification of the question "What should I expect from my doctor when first diagnosed?" This is a crucial time for you. We hope you received the examination, treatment, and care you needed and deserved at that time.

In order to give you an idea of what a first visit should involve, we consulted endocrinologist Dr. Michael Bush, director of the Diabetes Outpatient Training and Education Center at the Cedars-Sinai Medical Center in Los Angeles. He supplied a detailed account of what an ideal physical examination should be. (See Reference Section: Doctor's Initial Evaluation.)

After your first visit, you'll need to follow your doctor's recommendations for how often he or she wants to see you. It might be as frequently as three or four times a month at first. Once you get over your initial learning period and the doctor feels you're ready to be more independent, your visits may be cut down to once every three months, especially if he or she wants to order laboratory tests, such as a hemoglobin A_1C test. At each visit the doctor needs to check your testing records and go over your self-care with you to see where improvements and changes should be made. This is also your chance to ask any questions you've come up with since your last office visit.

Your doctor should also be available by telephone (or have a colleague who is available) at all times in case any serious diabetes-related emergency develops and you need help. The doctor should be willing to answer occasional questions by phone when you're having trouble handling some diabetes problem.

All this is just standard care, however. The more important expectations you should have deal with your doctor's attitudes and your interaction with him or her.

First and foremost, you should expect your doctor to treat you as an individual, not just a textbook diabetes case. You are a person with definite needs and interests and likes and dislikes, and they can and should be incorporated into your treatment. There are many different ways of handling diabetes—different diets, different exercise plans, different insulin-injection schedules that can make diabetes come at least halfway toward adjusting to your lifestyle.

In order for the doctor to make these variations on the basic theme of diabetes care, she or he is going to have to spend a little time finding out about you and your way of living, working, and playing. In other words, your doctor is going to have to talk to you. No, make that talk *with* you. There should be an interchange of ideas, not a lecture. The doctor should regard you as a colleague in your diabetes care and never convey the idea that you are incapable of understanding your condition and treatment. In fact, as Dr. Donnell B. Etzwiler says: "Diabetic patients provide 99 percent of their own care." So as your own physician you'd *better* be capable of understanding your condition and its treatment.

Your doctor, therefore, should give you a full explanation of all the laboratory tests you have. Rather than telling you your blood sugar is "normal" or "a little high, but still okay," he or she should tell you the exact figures. You should also know exactly where you stand with cholesterol, triglycerides, blood pressure—everything that affects your health and that you can make better or worse by your own behavior.

Now, although there are a lot of things that your doctor has to discuss with you, we don't want to lead you to expect that the doctor should have long, leisurely conversations with you, going over every facet of your physiological and psychological makeup. A doctor's time is too valuable to squander in great chunks. You are not the only patient, and others have their needs, too.

And speaking of time, *your* time has some value, too. You deserve a doctor who doesn't overbook and keep patients crouching in the waiting room for hours, building up stresses that are very bad for diabetes control.

This is not to say you should *never* have to wait. There are emergencies that a doctor must handle, and they can throw the schedule off, but if there is an emergency every time you have an appointment, you have cause for suspicion. We wouldn't carry on about waiting time to this extent except that since a diabetic goes to the doctor regularly every two or three months *forever,* that waiting-room time can really add up.

Since most doctors frankly admit that they lack a background in nutrition—one doctor told us he had had only a one-hour lecture on it during his entire time at medical school—you should expect your doctor to be able to refer you to a good dietitian to help you plan the complexities and personal variations of your diet. He or she shouldn't just throw a one-page diet list at you and send you on your way.

It is also extremely helpful if the office has a diabetes nurse specialist (a C.D.E.—certified diabetes educator) who can help you develop a good technique with injections, blood-sugar testing, diet, and problems of daily living. Again, these are specifics that the doctor doesn't have the time to help you with.

You should expect your doctor to keep up with the latest developments in the field of diabetes and be willing to incorporate them into your treatment.

Finally—and this may be asking too much—we personally feel that your doctor and other involved health professionals should also provide a good example. It's rather difficult for you to take good health advice from a flabby chain-smoker who is obviously ignoring all such counsel.

From all these "shoulds," you can see that it helps a great deal if your doctor is a diabetologist or an internist who specializes in diabetes.

How do I find a doctor who specializes in diabetes?

Doctors specializing in diabetes are usually listed under endocrinology and metabolism in the yellow pages. But rather than just sticking a pin in the telephone directory, you may prefer to call your local diabetes association and ask for the names of diabetologists who are closest to your home (and closeness *is* important). If your town has no local association, call your state affiliate of the American Diabetes Association and ask for a recommendation.

If you still have no luck, call your local hospital and ask who on their staff handles most of the diabetes cases.

Another good thing to do is go to your public library and check the *Directory of Medical Specialists.* This way you can find out the doctor's training, what hospitals he or she has worked in, age, and special experience. (This book is a little tricky to use. You may need to ask the librarian for help.)

We realize, however, that in some small towns there simply isn't a diabetologist. In that case, find (or keep) a doctor with whom you feel you can have a good relationship. Look for one who is willing to explore solutions to problems you present. Be sure she or he is willing to investigate new developments in diabetes that you may learn about in your reading or from discussions at meetings and seminars.

Incidentally, if you have a beloved family doctor, there's no reason to desert him or her for a diabetologist. You can keep the beloved one as your general physician and go to your diabetologist for special diabetes care.

When your diabetes is in its early stages or if you start developing problems at any time, you may want to go to one of the major diabetes clinics in the country where you stay a week or so and are given examinations and lab tests. You attend classes and learn what you need to do to get your diabetes under good control.

After all this talk about what your doctor should do for you, we mustn't forget your responsibilities to your doctor and what your doctor should expect from you.

What should my doctor expect from me?

Number one is honesty. Always tell the doctor the truth about what you're doing (or not doing) in your diabetes care. Report the true results of your blood-sugar tests. (One young woman told us she faked the results of the tests because she didn't want the doctor to be disappointed.) The doctor can't get you on the right track if he or she doesn't know that you're on the wrong one. Never try to fake the doctor out by behaving like a model diabetic for the few days just before you're scheduled for an examination and being very casual (sloppy) about your self-care the rest of the time.

You also owe your doctor cooperation. If you can't or won't follow the advice you're given, you should find another doctor whose advice you can and will accept.

Your doctor should also be able to expect you to take good care of yourself—not just your diabetes, but your *whole self.* Too many of us think we can neglect our health or even actively destroy it and then go to the doctor and say, "I'm sick. Make me well." Then if the doctor can't rectify the damage we've done, we get angry.

Don't take advantage of your doctor. If you phone constantly to discuss every little problem or try to monopolize his or her time in the office, using the doctor as a father or mother confessor, you're actually taking advantage of other patients whose time you're usurping.

It's ironic, but once you've found a doctor who is willing to listen, you have to be responsible enough to restrain yourself and stick to the facts of your diabetes problem. True, your personal problems *are* a part of the total picture of your diabetes, but a mention of their existence is enough. A diabetologist is not a psychiatrist and cannot be expected to straighten out your marriage, assuage your guilt feelings, release your inhibitions, or do whatever else is required to give you psychic peace.

If your life problems weigh unbearably upon you and you feel they are significantly detrimental to your diabetes control, ask your doctor to recommend a therapist to help you with them.

How much should I weigh?

A better question would be, What percentage of my body weight should be fat? The old height-weight-age tables are no longer considered good guides. Rather, correctness of weight should be determined by measuring the proportion of body fat and lean tissue. Simply weighing yourself is deceptive because muscle weighs more than fat, and it's the proportion of muscle to fat that counts from a health standpoint. In fact, you can be thin and still carry more fat than is healthy. When we sponsored a health-fair day at the Sugar-Free Center in Van Nuys, our thinnest employee—you can almost see through her—turned out to be too fat, and she was advised to lose some fat and build up more muscle. In fact, June, the only diabetic member of our Van Nuys staff at the time, was the only one who passed the test with flying colors. (It pays to be a well-disciplined diabetic.)

The recommended proportion of body fat is different for men and women. Men should be between 6 and 23 percent fat and women between 9 and 30 percent, depending on age. Men who are 25 percent fat and women who are 35 percent fat are classified as obese. There is some controversy about these recommended figures, because this is a new concept, but since you already have diabetes as a risk factor it would seem wisest to play it safe and go for the lower end of the scale if at all possible (see Table 3).

In the first edition of this book we recommended a simple pinch test to see if you were too fat. You pinch up your flesh just below your ribs at your waistline. Pressing the flesh between your thumb and forefinger, you should find a thickness of between one-half and one inch. If the pinch test reveals more flesh than that, you're too fat.

A more precise way, one that will predict the exact percentage of fat, is a caliper test. This is done by taking pinches with a caliper at the midriff, on the chest, just below the shoulder, and on the front of the thigh. These results are averaged, and a table gives the corre-

TABLE 3.
Recommended Percent Body Fat

Age Group

Males	19–24	25–29	30–34	35–39	40–44	45–49	50–59	60+
Minimum (%)	6	6	6	6	6	6	6	6
Maximum (%)	14.8	16.5	18.0	19.4	20.5	21.5	22.7	23.5

Females								
Minimum (%)	9	9	9	9	9	9	9	9
Maximum (%)	21.9	22.4	22.7	23.7	25.4	27.2	30.0	30.8

Although there is no established "standard" for recommended percent body fat, this table is based on the consensus of many experts in the health field. (Copyright 1987, Futrex, Inc. Reprinted by permission)

sponding fat percentage. The caliper test must be taken in a doctor's office or at a fitness center.

The Futrex Company of Gaithersburg, Maryland, has an instant Body Fat Tester, the Futrex-100, which you simply place against your bicep and it displays your percent of body fat. It operates with an infrared beam (a certain wavelength is absorbed by fat but not by lean tissue). The price is around $100 (available from Self-Care Catalog, 1-800-345-3371).

The most accurate body-composition test is naturally the most awkward and expensive. For this, you need to be weighed underwater using a hydrodensitomer. Since fat floats and muscle sinks, the heavier you are underwater, the better. (It's the opposite of the situation on land.)

It seems to us that every diabetic should seek out a place to have one of these tests and find out his or her body composition. The tests are generally available at university medical centers, weight-loss clinics, health clubs, fitness centers, and some doctors' offices and sports-medicine centers. Incidentally, if you are overweight according to weight charts you could find out the happy news that your weightiness is mostly due to muscle and therefore not risky at all. In fact, researchers did a study that proved that overweight lean men have the same low risk of developing heart disease as normal-weight lean men. Only overweight fat men are at greater risk.

Do I have to worry about cholesterol?

Everyone these days is either worrying about cholesterol or worrying about whether they should be worrying about it. Still cholesterol is something you should take seriously, especially if you have diabetes. Diabetics are more likely to have higher levels of cholesterol and blood fats (triglycerides). It may be that high blood sugar causes elevation of LDLs (low-density lipoproteins, or "bad" cholesterol) and lowering of HDLs (high-density lipoproteins, or "good" cholesterol). HDLs are thought to remove cholesterol from the arteries, while LDLs lead to fatty deposits that clog the arteries and cause heart attacks.

Thus the American Diabetes Association's *Exchange Lists for Meal Planning* emphasizes eating vegetable fats (known as unsaturated fats). Vegetable fats do not contain dietary cholesterol; only animal fats do. The very best of the vegetable fats are the monounsaturated ones—avocado, canola, olive and peanut oils. Current recommendations are to eat no more than three hundred milligrams of cholesterol a day. There are books in which you can check the cholesterol content of different foods (see Recommended Reading).

The newest statistics from the National Cholesterol Education Program estimates that 52 million U.S. adults—29 percent—have cholesterol levels that are too high. Three-quarters of these people could correct their cholesterol levels with diet and exercise. The American Diabetes Association's recommended diet of 30 percent fat (10 percent of which may come from animal or saturated fat) is the ideal diet to keep cholesterol levels in check. Which is yet another reason being a diabetic puts you in the know about keeping healthy.

And what should your cholesterol level be? The consensus is that it should be under 200 milligrams of cholesterol per deciliter of blood; 240 is considered borderline high risk. It stands to reason that all diabetics should have regular cholesterol tests to make sure they stay under 200. It's best to be tested in your doctor's lab and not at those mass screenings in malls, which may not be accurate. Besides it's especially important to have your HDLs and LDLs checked at the same time. If you have below normal HDLs, you may be at risk, even though your total cholesterol is under 200. The ideal HDL level is over 50; ideal LDL is 130 or less. If you have enough HDLs you may not be at risk even though you are over 200.

As you've probably read in newspapers and magazines, oat bran is a potent reducer of blood cholesterol. Eating oat-bran cereal or oatmeal is the best way to take advantage of oat bran's cholesterol-lowering properties. Also, eat cold-water fish at least twice a week, because fish oils (omega-e fatty acids) lower cholesterol. And watch out for egg yolks; one = 270 mg of cholesterol.

Do I have to exercise?

A better question would be, Isn't it terrific that such an enjoyable activity as exercise is a basic part of diabetes therapy? The answer to both questions is yes.

Although exercise is often a neglected area in diabetes care, getting the right amount of exercise is just as important as following a good eating plan—if not more important.

We've heard it said that if you had to make a choice between eating junk food and exercising or eating a perfectly healthy diet and being immobile, you'd be healthier eating the junk food and exercising. Of course, you don't have to make that choice—in fact, you can't make it. You need both exercise and good food for optimum health and blood-sugar control.

Exercise is almost a magic formula for diabetics. If you're too thin—usually the lean, insulin-dependent types—it will help you gain needed pounds by causing you to utilize your food better. Since it acts like an "invisible insulin," it helps get glucose into the cells, so less is wasted by being spilled into the urine.

If you're overweight, exercise will help you lose weight—and keep it off. Contrary to the myth, exercise does *not* increase your appetite. In fact, it suppresses it by regulating your *appestat*, the brain center that controls the appetite, and redirecting the blood flow away from the digestive tract. As a result, you'll be able to eat more because of the calories you burn, and yet you'll feel like eating less. This combination will deliver you from that complaint of so many diabetics: "I'm always hungry."

Exercise also makes weight loss easier because it revs up your metabolism, with the result that you burn more calories even when you're sitting still or sleeping. This principle is explained in Covert Bailey's well-known book *The New Fit or Fat?*

Besides helping overweight Type II diabetics lose weight, exercise lowers blood sugar by actually increasing the number of insulin receptors—those cell "locks" that the key of insulin is inserted into.

Exercise helps all of you improve circulation and lower blood fats (cholesterol and triglycerides) and therefore helps ward off the heart and blood-vessel problems to which diabetics are subject.

The benefits of exercise are not limited to physical improvements. Exercise lessens stress and is a great mood elevator. Perhaps you've heard of those brain chemicals called endorphins. Endorphins are known as the morphine within and are released when you exercise. They give you a natural high such as runners experience after about a half hour. This kind of morphine is a drug worth getting hooked on.

The only tragedy associated with exercise is that of people who have physical problems that prevent them from doing it. Those of you who have proliferative retinopathy are warned that exercise may aggravate the problem. People with heart disease should also be aware of exercise cautions and check with their doctor before embarking on a program. And anyone with impaired circulation to the legs and feet should find out what precautions to take. Dr. Peter Lodewick, Chief Diabetologist Specialist, Diabetes Department, Eye Foundation Hospital in Birmingham, Alabama, says that such people should be particularly wary of getting blisters.

On a more encouraging note, we'd like to add that diabetes is no detriment to becoming an outstanding athlete. Some good examples are the tennis star Bill Talbert, the hockey player Bobby Clarke, and, in baseball, Jackie Robinson, Ron Santo, Bill Gullickson, and Catfish Hunter.

What kind of exercise should I do?

What kind of exercise do you like? Exercise should be fun. That's the only way to be sure you'll keep doing it. As a diabetic you have enough chores in your life without turning exercise into another one.

If you want to rate exercises, though, the ones that are best for you are the aerobic or endurance kind: brisk walking, jogging, running, swimming, cross-country skiing, biking (either on the real thing or, in bad weather, on an exercycle), rowing, jumping rope. Dancing is also a wonderful endurance exercise. There are now lots of aerobics classes designed especially to build up your cardiovascular system and endurance. Several television shows can lead you through a regular aerobic session, and you can buy videotapes to do the same.

But really, as we said, exercise is play and should be fun. Try to acquire a skill you enjoy, like tennis or bowling or golf, even if it isn't an endurance sport. We find that if you get really involved in a nonendurance sport, you tend to do some endurance exercising in order to—what else?—increase your endurance for the sport you love.

Yoga is also a wonderful exercise to keep you supple, and it's something that can be done at any age.

Be sure also to add to your activities some form of strengthening exercises. These are advocated by most experts now, because 60 percent of the body's muscles are above the hips. You can go a couple of times a week to a gym or fitness center (these also have aerobic equipment) and use Nautilus or Cybex strengthening equipment. Or simply work out at home with some weights.

You should have a minimum of three aerobic sessions a week of twenty to thirty minutes. Don't let more than two days elapse between workouts. It's better to exercise five times a week, and to our minds, exercising every day is the best, unless your body tells you not to, because then it's easier to balance your diet and medication. Incidentally, your blood sugar should be at least 150 before you begin your routine or you should eat a snack.

Your intensity goal should be to get your heart rate to between 60 and 65 percent of its maximum capacity. To figure your training pulse range, subtract your age from 220, then multiply the result by 60 percent. The 60 percent level is sufficient to promote fitness.

Before you begin an exercise program—and this is critical if you're out of shape—you should consult your physician and possibly have an exercise stress test. Your doctor may want to prescribe your individual heart target zone. And there is one instance in which exercise is harmful. If your blood sugar is 250 or over, exercise will simply run it higher and you may produce ketones.

The best time to exercise is after meals. This way, if you take insulin or oral drugs, you're less likely to get hypoglycemic. In fact, testing before, during, and after exercise is not a bad idea until you learn your blood-sugar pattern. You may need to lower your insulin or oral drug dosage or eat extra carbohydrate. Exercise has an effect on blood sugar for twenty-four hours. So watch for hypoglycemia (low blood sugar) the day after the exercise if you've done something special like a long hike or a day of skiing.

Type I's should not inject insulin into the parts of the body that will be most used during exercise. For instance, don't inject into your legs or the arm you'll use if you're going to play tennis. The insulin would be absorbed much faster than usual if you did.

Incidentally, don't let age stop you. Even if you have health problems in addition to diabetes, there is always some form of exercise you can practice. Almost everyone can at least start walking on a schedule and then increase distance and speed until it becomes an endurance exercise.

As well as getting into a regular exercise program and sports, it's important to bring more exercise into your daily life simply by becoming a more physically active person. Get up out of your chair and move whenever possible. Climb stairs rather than taking the elevator. Park your car in the farthest corner of the parking lot and walk to the store. (Since everybody else is always trying to get as close as possible, you'll get the dividend of not having your car dinged up by the other people opening their doors on it.)

Is joining a gym a good way to get exercise?

It can be if you really go and go regularly. If you are gregarious and like to work out in the company of others, a gym may be just the motivation you need. It's a good way to get acquainted with people who have the same interest in fitness that you do. You can inspire one another—and chide one another when you don't show up. Be sure to join a gym that's not too far from your home, though, or you'll wind up spending most of your exercise time on transportation or decide not to go at all.

Belonging to a gym also has the advantage of providing someone to watch over you when you exercise. It is important to tell people there that you're a diabetic and to explain what the symptoms of hypoglycemia are so they can spot them in the event you develop low blood sugar from exercise.

We heard peripatetic radio guru Bruce Williams say on one of his shows that when he belonged to a gym and got home from a trip, it was often too late to go to the gym or he was too tired to drive there, so he got himself a Schwinn Airdyne—an exercycle that exercises your arms as well as your legs. He said that when he got home "that darn thing was always there waiting for me and I had no excuses not to exercise." Purchasing your own exercise equipment and having it right at home might be a viable alternative for you. You could buy a new piece of equipment every year at about the cost of joining a gym (an Airdyne costs $600). If there are others in your household who could use the equipment, it makes it an even better deal. Don't worry if you don't have a place to put it. Exercise equipment is getting more compact and portable all the time. We have a friend who keeps her rowing machine behind the sofa in the living room. Barbara has a treadmill, a rebounder, and a rowing machine in her bedroom. This doesn't leave much space for anything else, and it doesn't enhance the decor, but health is more important than decor any day.

Walking is, of course, one of the best exercises of all, and it takes no equipment. It does have a few drawbacks, though: you can't do it in all weather, and in big cities the streets and parks are getting acutely hazardous, especially for women alone. For these reasons mall-walking is becoming a popular alternative.

So analyze yourself and choose whatever would be most likely to keep you exercising regularly. Then just do it. (P.S.: *Do it now.*)

What should I do if I'm always too tired to exercise?

To some extent, that depends on what you did to get tired. If you're weary from your job as steeplejack or longshoreman, or if you're a housewife who's cleaned the whole house or galloped after a four-year-old all day, you've already had a great deal of exercise. Getting more is not that critical for you.

On the other hand, if you're tired from a long day of sedentary office tensions or sitting in the car, you need exercise for more reasons than diabetic ones, and you should clamp your jaw and force yourself, at least initially. Just as the appetite comes with the eating, the energy and enthusiasm for exercise come with the exercising. Often the fatigue you feel at the end of the day comes from a *lack* of physical activity rather than from too much of it.

If you find yourself too tired to exercise and it's not a true physical tiredness, you may go to bed and find yourself too keyed up and tense to sleep. The next day you've got a lack-of-sleep tiredness going. Vicious cycle. But if you get out there and move those bones around, blessed sleep will descend upon you as soon as you hit the pillow. You'll sleep the sleep of the physically tired and virtuous. And you can hardly sleep a better sleep than that.

Will vitamins and minerals help my diabetes?

This question is as controversial as the question of whether vitamin and mineral pills do anybody any good. There are doctors who claim that the only thing these supplements do for most people is give them expensive urine. There are doctors who have a go-ahead-and-take-them-if-you-like attitude. And there are doctors who counsel their patients to take vitamin and mineral supplements to ensure that they aren't missing anything vital in their diet.

In theory, if you are eating the healthy, balanced, and varied diet you're supposed to, you're getting your vitamins in the best way possible—from the food you eat. However, since in diabetic diets calories are often limited, taking one standard multiple vitamin a day as a safety net seems like a sound idea. Women, of course, may need to take extra iron and calcium in certain cases, but usually your physician is aware of this and prescribes the proper type and dose.

Two minerals that are often touted as helping diabetics by improving insulin usage are zinc and chromium. So far, though, no scientific studies give conclusive results on either of them. Virginia

Valentine suggests, at least for Type II's, a mineral supplement of magnesium and chromium picolinate. Magnesium is lost from high blood sugars, diuretics and drinking coffee (it's taboo to take magnesium if you have a high creatinine level).

Recent recommendations are that all of us take antioxidants—vitamins C and E—because they protect against heart disease and cancer. Studies show that people with diabetes may have vitamin C deficiencies and that a dose of 1400 mg a day may improve their A_1C tests.

And finally, we're glad you asked "Will vitamins and minerals *help* my diabetes?" and not "Will vitamins and minerals *cure* my diabetes?" We, too, have read, in books of vitamin lore, fables of how diabetics were able to give up insulin injections entirely after loading up on vitamin supplements and health foods. Don't give yourself false hope. If you have surplus money, it's better to give it to research for a real cure for diabetes than to the vitamin industry for a false one.

What kind of eye problems can diabetes cause?

Blurred vision is one of the symptoms of long-term, out-of-control diabetes. After the diabetes is diagnosed and brought under control, vision usually returns to normal.

Because of the visual changes that can take place with changes in blood sugar, June's ophthalmologist always insists that she have normal blood sugar when she comes in to have her eyes checked to see if she needs new glasses.

When a diabetic suddenly has blurred vision or other strange visual happenings (June sometimes reports seeing a large spot of light in her field of vision), this can indicate low blood sugar. These changes in vision can be disturbing, but they don't mean you're going blind. Blindness is always a worry for diabetics because you hear so many horrendous statisics about it. Diabetes used to be the cause of blindness in 11 percent of the legally blind people in this country, making it the third leading cause of blindness. It is still the number-one cause of new cases of blindness in people under sixty-five.

The culprit in diabetic blindness is retinopathy. This is a damaging of the blood vessels in the retina, the light-sensitive area in the back of the eye. In its later stages the delicate blood vessels of the retina may develop tiny sacs that can burst and leak blood, causing a loss of vision.

This is one of the reasons your doctor always examines your eyes so carefully: to look for changes in your blood vessels. The retina is the one place in the human body where doctors can actually see and inspect the condition of the blood vessels. Not only is weakness in the walls of the retinal blood vessels bad news in itself, but the condition of these blood vessels reflects the condition of the vessels throughout the body. You see, eyes are not just the mirrors of the soul, as the poets say, but the mirrors of the body as well.

Retinopathy is one of the diabetic horribles that don't have to happen. The study published in February 1989 in the *Journal of the American Medical Association* showed that no diabetic who had good control (less than 1.1 times normal blood sugar) had *any* eye damage, whereas of those who had blood sugar consistently above 1.5 times normal, 37 percent had retinopathy. The DCCT confirmed this.

Even when retinopathy does develop, all is not lost. There has been a great deal of success in treating it with laser beams. As always, however, the best treatment is to keep your blood sugar normal and not develop the problem in the first place.

Why do they talk so much about diabetic foot care?

It's that same old vascular story. Diabetes can cause hardening and narrowing of the blood vessels. This, in turn, causes poor circulation of the blood. Since the feet are farthest away from the great blood pump, the heart, they get the worst deal. Poor blood circulation is also part of the aging process. So if you're older *and* diabetic, you've really got to watch those feet.

And we do mean *watch,* because if you also have a touch of neuropathy, you may not feel a cut, sore, blister, or ingrown toenail and let it go until it becomes infected. Infections are particularly hazardous because, combined with diminished circulation, they provide a welcome mat for gangrene (tissue destruction), which can necessitate amputation.

Here are the foot-care do's:

1. Wash your feet every day and wear clean socks.
2. Always dry well between your toes.
3. Cut your toenails after bathing, following the shape of the ends of the toes. Do not cut too short.
4. Wear well-fitting shoes.
5. Examine your feet daily for signs of infection.
6. If you develop foot problems, go to a podiatrist and tell him or her you are diabetic. In fact, we favor regular visits to a podiatrist.

Here are the foot-care don'ts:

1. Avoid elastic garters or anything tight around the legs or ankles.
2. Do not use heating pads or hot-water bottles on your feet.
3. Avoid smoking; it reduces the blood supply to the feet.
4. Never walk around barefoot.
5. Do not use corn plasters or any over-the-counter foot medications.
6. Do not cut corns and calluses.
7. Do not put your feet in water warmer than eighty-five or ninety degrees Fahrenheit.

If you need convincing to make you behave yourself in the foot department, the Loma Linda Diabetes Education Program offers the story of a man who didn't take care of his diabetes *or* his feet. As he aged and deteriorated, he lost his sight and all feeling in his feet. Well, it came to pass that one night, without knowing it, he knocked his watch off his bedside table and into his shoe and broke the crystal. He walked around on said broken watch for two weeks. Needless to say, he wound up as a guest in the Loma Linda Hospital.

If you are a middle-aged or older diabetic, you should watch for symptoms of diminished circulation: weak pulses in the feet and legs; cold, dry, pale skin on the feet and legs; lack of hair growth on the toes; and toes that turn a dusky red color when they hang down, as when you're sitting on the edge of the bed. Be sure to mention it to your doctor if you notice any of these symptoms.

It is possible to improve or maintain the circulation in your feet with a simple exercise. Lie on a bed with your feet raised above your hips. Alternate pointing your toes and heels toward the ceiling. Do this several times. Make circles with your feet, first clockwise, then counterclockwise. Sit up with your feet hanging over the edge of the bed. Repeat the same maneuvers as above. Do this exercise a couple of times a day.

When you get your feet in good shape, walking a mile or more daily in comfortable shoes (runners' training shoes are good) can be of great benefit.

We don't want to give the impression that older diabetics are the only ones who have to be careful of their feet. Although younger people generally have better circulation, they still can get into trouble especially if their diabetes is out of control.

Is there anything special I should do about my teeth?

If you're under good control, you'll treat your teeth as everyone is supposed to—daily flossing at night, brushing away the plaque at gum level after meals, regular visits to your dentist for removal of tartar (hardened plaque), and any other routines recommended for you personally. But if you have continual high blood sugars, your mouth, especially your gums, will be in jeopardy. The sad truth is that diabetes is sometimes diagnosed by a dentist because its damaging effects show up in your mouth.

What the dentist may see when inspecting the teeth of an individual who has undiagnosed or uncontrolled diabetes is periodontal (gum) disease. This is an inflammation of the gums and bone around the teeth caused by bacteria. Plaque is a soft accumulation of this bacteria. Plaque makes your gums bleed and eventually pull away from the teeth, forming open pockets that can deepen until you lose teeth.

Diabetes also lowers your mouth's ability to deter the bacterial infection. Bleeding gums are a sign of periodontal problems, as is bad breath. It pays, though it's expensive, to go to your dentist regularly, because periodontal disease and other oral infections can make blood-sugar control more difficult. It's the old vicious circle.

I have pain in my feet. My doctor says this is neuropathy. What is neuropathy?

Since the first edition of this book in 1981 we have received more letters about this complication of diabetes than any other. Simply put, neuropathy is nerve damage caused by high blood glucose. The most common type is "peripheral neuropathy," which means it affects the nerves in the feet, legs, and hands. Feet are the main source of complaint for most people.

The symptoms of neuropathy are described as pins and needles, tingling, numbness, or burning pain. You can even have complete loss of sensation. When this happens to your feet, it's very dangerous, because you won't be aware of blisters or injuries, or even of stepping on a tack.

Another form of neuropathy, "autonomic," affects the internal organs—stomach, urinary tract, small blood vessels, and even the genitals (this can cause impotence in men). Though generally not painful, this kind of nerve damage leads to serious disorders with the digestion (gastroparesis or slow emptying of the stomach), diarrhea or constipation, and unawareness of insulin reactions.

Treatments for all types of neuropathies start with bringing blood sugar under control. This alone can reverse the damage by as much as 50 percent in beginning cases. The strange phenomenon is that sometimes at first your discomfort becomes greater and lessens only after several months of normal blood sugars.

In cases of severe pain and gastrointestinal problems your doctor can prescribe various drugs. For peripheral neuropathy a cream called Zostrix (over-the-counter) or the three-times-stronger Axsain (by prescription) have proven effective for many people but they often have to be used regularly for several weeks before you notice any improvement. Both these creams contain capsaicin, derived from chili peppers, so keep your fingers away from your eyes after applying it.

Researchers are now studying the use of a family of drugs called "aldose-reductase inhibitors" to treat mild cases of neuropathy. If the clinical trials are successful, these drugs may be of great benefit to sufferers.

Why do they say people with diabetes heal much slower than normal?

They say that because they don't differentiate between people in control (mostly normal blood sugars) and those out of control (mostly high blood sugars). If you are an in-control person, don't let health professionals prejudice you against yourself in this way. This is what Deepak Chopra, M.D., author of *Quantum Healing,* calls a *nocebo,* a term which denotes the opposite effect of a placebo. A nocebo is a negative effect caused by a doctor's opinion or prediction. If in a doctor's office you are told, "You won't heal very fast because of your diabetes," block out that thought and if you have a good A_1C, tell yourself instead that your healing time will be normal or faster.

Testimonial: June once had a hand surgery (nothing to do with diabetes) and the orthopedic surgeon volunteered the statement, "You healed faster than most people."

Is it all right to use hot tubs?

According to the U.S. Consumer Product Safety Commission, all people who have diabetes, a history of heart disease, or blood-pressure problems should check with a doctor on the advisability of using a hot tub.

They also caution that nobody should bathe in a hot tub with water that is 104 degrees Fahrenheit or higher, since water of 106 degrees Fahrenheit can be fatal even to fully healthy adults. (Barbara, who considers herself a fully healthy adult, gets rather frightening nosebleeds after sitting in Japanese baths or hot springs.)

The preceding section on foot care explains that you shouldn't put your feet in water warmer than 85 or 90 degrees Fahrenheit. Since it's a little awkward to soak in a hot tub with your feet hanging out, it looks as if tepid tubs should be the order of the day for diabetics.

I have a bad case of acne. Could this be caused by my diabetes?

Possibly. Some diabetics report that they have acne when their diabetes is out of control and that it clears up when their blood sugar is stabilized.

Then again, it's possible that your acne has nothing to do with your diabetes. Many diabetics have a tendency to figure that every physical problem from acne to Zenker's diverticulum of the esophagus is related to their diabetes. When June had chronic headaches, she at first thought they were caused by low blood sugar. It turned out they had nothing to do with diabetes.

It is true that diabetes, especially out-of-control diabetes, can cause a variety of minor and not-so-minor health problems. Still, you should try to avoid laying the blame for everything on diabetes. Not only does this make you feel more depressed and put upon, but it may also cause you to delay seeking treatment for whatever your problem really is.

Are flu shots necessary?

They don't always work because there are often so many different strains of flu going around that you get zapped by one your shot doesn't cover. Still, we think they're a good idea. Flu can upset control of blood sugar for insulin takers, and flu shots are usually recommended for older people. Put those two groups together and you've just about covered the whole diabetic population.

Since flu shots themselves can cause rather heavy flu symptoms in susceptible beings, it's sometimes wise to take two half doses at different times. June always does this with flu shots and with shots she has to take for foreign travel as well.

Why do doctors always insist that you give up smoking?

Smoking is dangerous for everyone, but doubly dangerous for diabetics. Inhaling cigarette smoke affects the blood vessels. Diabetes can affect the blood vessels. Both diabetes and smoking tend to narrow them, and narrowed arteries can cause heart disease and gangrene.

An out-of-control diabetic has 2.5 times the normal chances of getting heart disease. A smoker has 1.7 times the normal chances of dying of heart disease. Put the two together and you have over 4 times the normal risk of heart disease.

An out-of-control diabetic has 60 times the normal chances of getting gangrene of the feet. Again, smoking increases that already dismal figure.

A study done at the University Hospital in Copenhagen, Denmark, found that diabetic patients who smoked required 15 to 20 percent more insulin than nonsmokers. Their level of blood fats was also higher.

You might call smoking a kind of Virginia roulette for diabetics. So why are there diabetic smokers? That's a question we have no answer for, except that their use of nicotine is an addiction harder to kick than an addiction to heroin. So people try and fail and try and fail ad infinitum.

The best suggestion we have is to seek help. Without help, your chance of quitting (and not relapsing) is slim indeed. A government survey found that only about 10 percent of the smokers who want to quit seek help. That is thought to be the reason why so few succeed.

Where can you get help? Many hospitals now have clinics or treatment centers specializing in smoking-cessation programs. There are independent programs too, like Smokenders and Schick. Ask your doctor for advice. Just be sure the system you try addresses all the dependency problems of smoking: the physical, the psychological, and the social. As Dr. Judith Ockene, director of preventive and behavioral medicine at the University of Massachusetts Medical Center, pointed out in a *New York Times* article, "the most effective methods deal with a smoker's three-pronged dependency and recognize that quitting is a process—not a one-time event—that occurs three or four times over five to ten years."

DIABETES AND YOUR DAILY LIFE

Should I tell people I have diabetes?

In general, definitely yes. You should tell everyone you have any kind of regular, everyday contact with—your hairdresser or barber, your colleagues at work, your teachers, your coaches, your friends (even rather casual ones), and especially those with whom you play sports.

You should make it a special point to tell anyone with whom you have any kind of medical and semimedical dealings, such as your dentist or podiatrist or oculist, because that may influence their treatment of you.

There are several good reasons for letting people know you have diabetes, especially if you are insulin-dependent. In the first place, should you have an insulin reaction, a person in the know can help you out or at least will realize that whatever is happening to you may be related to your diabetes and will get you to someone who can help.

You are also much less likely to inadvertently offend people if they know you have diabetes. For example, if you get low blood sugar and suddenly turn into a grouch or hellion, they may realize it's because of your diabetes, not because of a mean streak that's part of your nature. Then, too, if you're eating at a friend's house and turn down a sugar-shot confection, the cook will know that you're not insulting his or her culinary talents but just behaving yourself and dutifully following your own diabetic diet.

Another reason for informing people about your diabetes is that you can help out others by educating nondiabetics as to what diabetes is. What those with diabetes need is an each-one-teach-one program in order to spread diabetes facts and wipe out some of those weird fictions that are floating around in the public mind, such as, "People with diabetes can't eat sugar, but they can eat all the honey they want because honey is natural."

If you do tell others about your diabetes, you're also likely to find that you are not as alone in your condition as you thought. Almost everyone you mention your diabetes to will start telling you about a diabetic cousin or grandmother—or even about their diabetic selves!

As part of your diabetes announcement program, you should certainly wear some sort of identification bracelet or medallion. This is a safeguard in case you are ever in an accident or have some kind of diabetic problem when you're away from those who know you. A particularly good identification is a Medic Alert bracelet (available from Medic Alert Foundation, Turlock, California 95381-1009, 1-800-ID ALERT). Medic Alert is well known now, and ambulance attendants, members of the ski patrol, and nurses in emergency hospitals are on the lookout for its insignia.

Now, after advocating this policy of extreme honesty, we'll hedge a bit. You don't have to be obsessed with your diabetes and immediately tell everyone you meet, "Hello-there-I'm-John-Smith-and-I'm-diabetic-pleased-to-meet-you," any more than you'd announce to a new acquaintance that you have gallstones or are color-blind or wear a pacemaker. As you get to know people better, your diabetes will emerge appropriately and naturally as a subject for conversation.

As for telling prospective employers and insurance agents, it's a yes-and-no situation that we'll discuss shortly.

Which is the correct thing to say: "I am a diabetic" or "I have diabetes"?

Do you mean correct or *politically* correct? Actually either is correct. As Lois Jovanovic-Peterson, M.D., wrote in *The Diabetic*

Woman, "I always say that it doesn't matter if I am a person with syphilis or a syphilitic—I still have the same disease." The same holds true with diabetes. Several years ago *Diabetes in the News* ran a reader survey to see which was the preferred way. "I am a diabetic" won a clear victory. Most people thought it was more straightforward and more accepting of your condition.

But then was then and times have changed. If you want to be politically correct now, that's a different matter. There's a growing movement to never use "diabetic" as a noun. The American Diabetes Association forbids its use in any of its publications. (On the other hand, we heard a radio ad for the Juvenile Diabetes Foundation in which they referred to "diabetics.")

We frequently get letters from people who range from wounded to furious when they're called "a diabetic." They feel that saying "I am a diabetic" gives the disease primary importance in your life, whereas saying "I have diabetes" or referring to "a person with diabetes" shows the disease to be of only secondary importance. Your individual personhood is what counts. And they certainly have a point.

June, call-a-spade-a-spade person that she is, has always referred to herself as "a diabetic," and you can see from the title of this book and the frequent reference to "diabetics" that we use the term interchangeably with the other more acceptable forms. But we don't like to gratuitously offend or hurt people to whom what they're called and call themselves makes a big difference. We tried to get the publisher to change the title of this book to *The Diabetes Book: All Your Questions Answered,* but that didn't fly because, since this is a new edition of a previously published book, you can't change the title in midstream. We have, however, changed the title of the next book we're writing from The *Diabetic's Good Times Therapy Book* to *The Diabetes Good Times Therapy Book.*

And, although you may not believe it when you see the number of times we still use "diabetic and diabetics" as nouns in this new edition, we *have* made a concerted effort to be more sensitive to those who are offended by that usage. It's just that in order to keep the cost of production of the book (and, therefore, the price to the consumer) down, we weren't always able to change "diabetic" into "person with diabetes" when there were no other substantive changes to be made on that page or where there just wasn't space for the extra two words.

The pendulum, however, may be swinging back. In July 1993 the National Federation of the Blind adopted a resolution (#93-01) condemning all euphemisms for blind ("people with blindness," "visually impaired") and declaring that it is respectable to be blind and there is no shame in it.

But whether you use the approved or unapproved diabetes term, either way will make you easily understood. Just don't shy away from both terms and use something cryptic the way June did once on a flight to Hawaii, when she was trying to get her meal from the flight attendant. "I'm on insulin," she said. "Could you serve me first?" The answer was negative. The problem, we figured out later, was that the flight attendant, who was Danish, didn't have any idea what June was talking about. In fact, she probably thought that insulin was the name of some kind of group tour of the islands and that June was just trying to get a special privilege for no good reason.

When Barbara trotted back a few minutes later and made eyeball-to-eyeball contact with the flight attendant and announced, "My friend is a di-a-bet-ic (that's the way she said it back in those days!) and she needs to eat. Could you serve her now?" the meal appeared a few seconds faster than immediately.

Now on to the question of the grammar of the words *diabetic* and *diabetes.* Experts have very definite ideas about correctness in the use of the words *diabetes* and *diabetic.* They don't like you to use *diabetic* as an adjective, unless what you're talking about actually has diabetes. For example, "The diabetic man had a diabetic dog" is all right, because both the man and the dog are diabetics. "The diabetic education lecture was held at the diabetic study center" is all wrong, because neither the education lecture nor the study center has diabetes. It should be "The diabetes education lecture was held at the diabetes study center."

You wouldn't say "a diabetic specialist" unless the specialist you're talking about has diabetes. If he's a specialist in diabetes, he should be called a diabetes specialist. If he's a specialist in diabetes who has diabetes, then presumably he'd be referred to as a "diabetic diabetes specialist." But maybe you think this is being linguistically nitpicky. Maybe we think so, too.

Just to put the capper on the whole nomenclatural confusion, the British call their organization the British Diabetic Association. But they always did have trouble with the language.

Will I be able to get insurance?

That depends on the kind of insurance you're interested in getting.

Automobile insurance. There should be no trouble if you're in good control. (Here's yet another reason to take good care of yourself.) If they ask on the form if you're a diabetic, naturally you have to tell them. In that case, they'll probably ask you to produce a letter from your doctor saying that your diabetes is under control.

If they don't ask, we don't see any point in saying "Hey there, insurance company, I have diabetes. Don't you want to hassle me?" Personal experience: June's automobile insurance company has never asked; she has never told.

Life insurance. If you're in control (again with evidence required) and you take less than forty units of insulin—or don't take insulin at all—you should have no more difficulty getting life insurance than a nondiabetic. We have, however, heard of cases in which people working for very small companies were denied both life insurance and disability insurance coverage on company policies.

Health Insurance. We don't need to tell you that this is the big can of worms as far as people with diabetes are concerned. Actually it's more like a can of snakes since it's such a hazardous and potentially lethal situation.

In every update on health insurance we write for people with diabetes, we keep hoping that we'll be able to say things are improving. So far there has been no improvement. In fact, things seem to be getting worse, as during a period of economic stress, companies try to cut costs by laying off employees and reducing benefits to remaining employees and retirees while the government is looking for any way it can to put a lid on ever-escalating health-care costs, especially for Medicare and Medicaid.

Oh, yes, we know that health-care reform in which all Americans will be adequately covered "is just around the corner," but this corner is a lot like the one that the cure for diabetes is just around. The corner never seems to get turned.

When President Clinton was campaigning for election, he said he'd announce a health-care plan in his first one hundred days in office. Then it was pushed to June, then to September. As of this writing, predictions are that even when the plan is announced, there will be five to seven years of special-interest wrangling and Congressional waffling before anything is in place. In the meantime the situation for unemployed or self-employed people with diabetes and those whose employers don't provide insurance is rapidly going from difficult to impossible.

Writer Alice Furlaud, in a commentary about her diabetes on the National Public Radio program "All Things Considered," departed from her usual lighthearted style to paint a picture that by comparison makes van Gogh's dark and dismal *Potato Eaters* look like a Breughel painting of carefree revelry. She explained that as a freelance writer she has to pay for all of her insurance herself. The premium for that insurance is over $5,000 a year, and she's been warned that it may go up again. And for all that money, this is what her insurance does for her:

"Last year I claimed $754.97 in medical expenses which, after the $300 deductible, came to $454.97, of which I am supposed to pay 20 percent, leaving $363.98 to be refunded by the insurance company. They have refunded precisely $77.03."

Not only that, but if she doesn't pay her quarterly payment right on the dot, she gets letters threatening to cut her insurance off. But when they owe her money, "they take a long time to pay; often they do not pay a cent."

She says this expensive health insurance "is dangerous to my health." Because of the cost of the insurance and the meager amount they pay, she hasn't been able to go to a gynecologist or eye doctor for years. The one time she went to a diabetes clinic, the cost of having a few blood tests and seeing a specialist for fifteen minutes was $600. The insurance company reimbursed her only $230. In the commentary she said that her quarterly payment of $1,327.54 was due and, "I just don't know how I'm going to pay it."

Three months later we read a travel article in the *New York Times* by Ms. Furlaud. The author identification said that she was based in Paris, where she was researching a book. Maybe she should do as Robert and Suzanne Massie did and tap into the French health-care system. Their son has hemophilia, and in her book, *Journey*, Suzanne said that when her husband was writing his book, *Nicholas and Alexandra*, they lived in Paris. One of the reasons they moved there was that the French government took care of their son's disease. In America, there was no help and no way for them to afford it themselves.

Although there are more unknowns than knowns in what the future holds for health insurance in America, one thing is pretty certain. More and more people will be with HMOs than ever before, since that's the most cost-effective way to deliver health care. One of the ways they keep costs lower is that you have to go through a "gatekeeper" doctor before you can see a specialist. And there are often limits to what they will do for you, usually financial limits.

As you can see from the following table, which appeared in *Diabetes Interview*, the kind of intensive diabetes therapy recommended by the DCCT to prevent complications is expensive.

Will HMOs be willing to pay these increased costs? That remains to be seen. One iconoclastic doctor we talked to at the ADA conference, where the DCCT results were announced, said it will probably take a few lawsuits from people who developed complications as a result of having the proven-effective intensive therapy denied them by their HMOs.

One bright note in this *symphonie pathétique* is that certain insurance companies are starting to reimburse for diabetes education conducted by ADA-recognized programs. This seeming realization that it's a good business practice to help people prevent complications rather than to pay for the much more expensive treatments for them later on down the line may make dramatic changes on both the insurance and HMO scenes.

Diabetes Interview Estimate

Treatment Method	Conventional Therapy *(using injections)*	Intensive Therapy *(using multiple injections)*	Intensive Therapy *(using an insulin pump)*
Shots/Day	2	4	continuous
Insulin & Syringe or Infusion Set	44¢	88¢	$3.66
Pump Cost/Day	—	—	$2.67
Blood Tests/Day	2	8	8
Strip Cost (72¢ ea.)	$1.44	$5.80	$5.80
Supply Cost/Month	$101	$247	$368.96
Supply Cost/Year	$1,208*	$2,960*	$4,427.45*

*Includes $125 meter, cost spread over 2 years. Pump therapy includes $3,900 pump, cost spread over 4 years.

(Reprinted from *Diabetes Interview*. For more information call 1-800-473-4636.)

We hope that more such positive changes will be made so all people with diabetes can have effective and affordable care without having to move to Paris or develop complications and sue. But one thing is certain. Just as Joan Hoover says in *The Dragon Diabetes* (see Reference Section), a cure for diabetes won't come about unless we, personally, all work hard and exert pressure on those who are in control of the situation, and neither will health-care reform. It's up to us. Are we up to it?

Will diabetes keep me from getting a job?

It didn't keep actress Mary Tyler Moore, radio and TV personality Gary Owens, hockey star Bobby Clarke, prominent physician Peter Forsham, or McDonald's restaurant tycoon Ray Kroc from getting the jobs they wanted. Why would it keep you from any career you choose? The truth is that the great majority of people with diabetes have the same employment opportunities and limitations as non-diabetics. So if you're qualified for a particular position, go after it positively and aggressively, and with confidence. Studies have shown that having diabetes promotes not only a healthy life-style but also great self-discipline. These in turn lead to superior performance on the job.

We have two examples of young men seeking their heart's choice of career—to be a doctor—in spite of being Type I diabetics. Their experiences also demonstrate the difference between then and now, between the old days of prejudice and discrimination against diabetics and the new ones of open opportunity.

Then

George L. Chappell, M.D., a psychiatrist practicing in Ventura, California, has been a diabetic for over thirty-seven years now. He knew from the age of four that he wanted to be a physician, so he actually overqualified himself during high school and college: high grades, a job, community volunteer service, everything to show he could succeed and carry a heavy workload. He applied to twenty medical schools and was rejected by all of them. One admissions officer told him: "Well, George, your qualifications are certainly way above average, but you're not going to live long enough for society to regain the investment that it makes in your education, so we won't be able to accept you." But Dr. Chappell persisted, pulling every string he could until finally the admissions officer at the University of California at Los Angeles caved in. He is still very much alive and has found the struggle well worth it, as "the emotional and professional rewards are great." He says that because of diabetes, he has a degree of empathy and personal experience that physically healthy physicians lack. Many of his patients notice his special concern and are grateful to have found such an out-of-the-ordinary therapist.

Now

Our first employee at the original SugarFree Center in Van Nuys, California, Ron Brown, joined us the summer before he planned to enter a Ph.D. program in psychology. As a diabetic himself, he had an instant rapport with all of our clients and, because of his deep reading in the field of diabetes, was invaluable in providing support and counseling.

The warm feelings that our clients felt toward Ron were obviously reciprocated. He soon knew that he wanted to devote his life to working with diabetics. Because of his talent for gourmet cooking and because he saw the difficulty most diabetics have in understanding and adjusting to the dietary changes their disease requires, he decided to work toward his R.D. degree.

After his swift and successful completion of the R.D. program at the University of California at Berkeley, he came back to work with us at the Del Mar, California, SugarFree Center and served as a dietitian at the nearby Scripps Clinic. His increased experience in diabetes at Scripps and with us heightened his interest in the field and made him realize that to do as much as he wanted to do to help others with diabetes, he would have to become a physician. Therefore, on top of working both at Scripps and at the SugarFree Center, he took the additional premed courses he lacked.

Ron applied for entrance to medical school in 1986 at the age of thirty. Both his age and his diabetes could have worked against him. Neither did. He was accepted by three medical schools without a quibble and probably would have been accepted by more except that he withdrew his other applications when he was accepted at the one he really wanted, the University of California at Davis. He now has his M.D. and is doing his three years of residency. June is looking forward to having him as her doctor in the very near future.

Not only does Ron's story show that prejudices against diabetes in the work world are crumbling, but it poses an interesting question. Would he be where he is today—getting ready to embark on a medical career—if he had not developed diabetes? As our former nurse-educator, Elsie Smallback, always said, "Out of something bad comes something good."

Ron's story reminds us of what we read about prize-winning novelist Walker Percy. He had gone to medical school because it was the thing to do in his family. After graduation he decided to go into psychiatry and interned at Bellevue Hospital in New York. He never practiced, though, because he contracted pulmonary tuberculosis and spent three years recuperating. For much of that time he was flat on his back, reading voraciously, mostly fiction and philosophy, which ultimately led to his literary career. He calls tuberculosis "the best disease I ever had. If I hadn't had it, I might be a second-rate shrink practicing in Birmingham at best."

Some years from now, it will be interesting for you to muse awhile on how your life has changed *for the better* because of your diabetes. You may well be surprised at what you come up with.

Realistic optimists that we are, however, we do have to report a few—very few—negatives in career selection for diabetics who take insulin. You should avoid jobs where you could endanger yourself or others during insulin reactions. It wouldn't be wise for you to seek jobs that involved high-speed machinery or climbing around on skyscraper construction girders, for example. Legally, there are certain restrictions, too. The federal government does not allow diabetics on insulin to enter the armed forces, to pilot airplanes, or to drive trucks or buses in interstate commerce, though there is a three-year moratorium on this last stipulation while the Federal Highway Administration assesses how Type I's perform.

If you should run into job discrimination because of diabetes, don't hesitate to fight it. Federal regulations have made it illegal for most major employers to reject you solely because you have diabetes. The Americans with Disabilities Act, which considers diabetes legally a disability, gives you the option of filing a complaint if you experience discrimination in the workplace. Employers cannot even ask you if you have diabetes during a job interview and must make reasonable accommodation for your diabetes needs.

FOR MEN:
Will my diabetes cause sexual problems?

According to early statistics, between 40 and 60 percent of diabetic men are ultimately affected by impotence. (A variation on this statistical theme is that the incidence of impotence is 15 percent in diabetic men between the ages of thirty and forty and 55 percent by age fifty.) As Mark Twain said, "There are lies, damned lies, and statistics." These statistics are probably akin to the now false figures about how many diabetics go blind or have amputations and kidney failure—all computed from the period when we didn't have the therapies we now have to keep blood sugar normal.

We actually hate to even quote these impotence statistics since reading them is just the sort of thing that could cause it. One psychologist we heard at a conference recounted the story of one of his patients who wasn't aware of the existence of diabetic impotence and was getting along just fine. When he heard the discouraging word, it was instant impotence for him. So if you're not having any problems in that line and if you're keeping your blood sugar normal, forget the statistics and go on with your life—and your sex life. If you've had or are having some problems or harbingers thereof, read on.

First of all, the impotence legends reflect several factors. Sometimes when a man is an undiagnosed, out-of-control diabetic, he can develop a *temporary* impotence, which goes away when his diabetes is diagnosed and he gets his blood sugar back in the normal range. This has inflated the statistics cited above.

Second, when diabetes is first diagnosed, a man is shot with so many negative emotions—such as anxiety, depression, anger, guilt, fear of rejection, and worry over his future—that he becomes impotent for psychological reasons, not because of his diabetes.

Sometimes the problem is caused by what sex therapists William H. Masters and Virginia E. Johnson call "spectatoring." Raul C. Schiavi and Barbara Hogan, writing in *Diabetes Care,* vividly describe the situation in which a diabetic man has heard the statistics and wonders if he's going to be a victim of them: "The diabetic patient, rather than becoming involved in the sexual experience and abandoning himself into erotic sensations and feelings, may find himself constantly monitoring the state of his penis. He becomes a witness rather than a participant in the sexual experience." Not surprisingly, this "performance anxiety" often results in impotence.

Indeed, the *British Medical Journal* reported that diabetic impotence was most likely caused by psychological factors in two-thirds of the men studied and by physical factors in only one-third. On the other hand, the brochure of the Recovery of Male Potency Program at Grace Hospital in Detroit says, "Twenty years ago, most doctors thought that impotence was primarily a psychological problem. We now realize that 80 percent of impotence has a physical rather than a psychological cause." And Ginger Manley, R.N., M.S.N., writing in the *Diabetes Educator,* states, "While in the general population only about 50 percent of impotence is physical in origin, in the diabetic population physically mediated impotence approaches 90 percent." (You read your statistics and you take your choice.) In short, impotence can be a combination of physical and psychological factors.

An easy and inexpensive way for you to determine if impotence is psychological or physical has been suggested by the broadcaster-columnist Dr. Gabe Mirkin. He explains that there are two stages of sleep: rapid-eye-movement (REM) and non-rapid-eye-movement sleep. In non-rapid-eye-movement sleep, males achieve an erection. This can occur several times throughout the night, and the male wakes up the next morning without even knowing it happened.

If you are achieving erections in the night, your impotence is psychological. To check this out, Dr. Mirkin recommends taking a roll of postage stamps (the one-cent kind, for thrift's sake), tearing off the appropriate number of stamps (he suggests four), and securing them tightly to the penis before going to bed. If the stamps are torn apart in the morning, you know you're having erections.

To make sure that anxiety resulting in fitful sleep doesn't confuse the issue, it might be a good idea to try this test more than once before deciding that your impotence is physical rather than psychological.

What can I do about impotence that is mainly psychological?

We hope it will help some just to have the reassurance that it *is* mainly psychological and that when you start handling the negative emotions that engulfed you with your diagnosis of diabetes, the sex problem will gradually disappear.

We know, however, that such emotions and their effects can't always be swept away with logic and Dutch-uncle conversations with yourself. You can't immediately eliminate your problem just because you've been told what's causing it. It takes time and consideration (consideration of yourself by yourself as well as consideration from your partner). If it takes too much time—and only you can decide how much is too much—you shouldn't hesitate to get some psychological help.

If your doctor isn't able to recommend a psychological counselor or sex therapist, you can contact any large university in your area. Most of these have human-sexuality programs and can give you the names of qualified sex therapists who are available for private consultation. And it is imperative that both you and your partner go to the therapist.

What can I do about impotence that is caused by physical factors?

Richard K. Bernstein, M.D., in his book *Diabetes: The Gluco-graF™ Method for Normalizing Blood Sugar,* suggests that if impotence in Type I diabetics is occasional and if it occurs during the first five to ten years of the disease, the "inability to become aroused or, if aroused, inability to achieve orgasm can be an early warning of hypoglycemia [low blood sugar]. . . . This early warning sign has been detected by both males and females. In fact, patients have located the blood-sugar levels at which they 'turn off.' " He continues, "It appears that both men and women tend to have two turnoff points: at one blood-sugar level they can be aroused but cannot achieve orgasm; at a lower blood-sugar level they cannot even be aroused. . . . Some patients try to prevent an unpleasant situation by measuring blood sugar when feasible prior to anticipated intercourse and promptly take fast-acting sweets if blood sugar is low."

You can also become impotent while under the influence of certain drugs. Among these are alcohol, tranquilizers, and marijuana. In many older men, impotence may be caused by hypertension drugs, with diabetes getting the blame. When possible, these suspect drugs should be avoided or their use discontinued. Your physician may be able to suggest an alternative medication.

Most long-range, gradually occurring impotence in diabetics is due to one or a combination of three factors:

1. a decrease in the male hormone, testosterone. This is the least likely of the three. It can be treated with hormone injections.

2. an interruption of the blood flow to the penis, usually as a result of atherosclerosis (hardening of the arteries).

3. neuropathy—damage to the nerves that carry the sexual message from the brain and dilate the blood vessels. This neuropathy is usually caused by long-term poor control of blood sugar and is sometimes reversible with improved control.

Some treatments that have proved successful include injections of drugs that improve the supply of blood to the penis, the use of vacuum-constriction devices, and penile implants. The implants can be rigid, semirigid, or inflatable. Anyone seeking help with physiological impotence should consult with a urologist. There are also many hospitals now setting up impotency programs where the problem of impotence can be evaluated, the options explained, and corrective procedures instituted. These programs often include invaluable support groups.

For background reading on diabetic impotence and its treatment, there is the "Sexual Man" chapter in the book *The Diabetic Man* by Peter Lodewick, M.D. There is also an excellent article, "Diabetes and Sexual Health," by Ginger Manley, R.N., M.S.N., in Vol. 12, No. 4, of *The Diabetes Educator*. If you can't find it in a local library, write to the American Association of Diabetes Educators (see Reference Section). For more good information send a stamped, self-addressed, legal size envelope with $1 for handling to the nonprofit Impotence Institute of America, 119 S. Ruth St., Maryville, TN 37801. Phone: (615) 983-6064.

It's important to remember that with impotence, as with all problems associated with diabetes, the best treatment is no treatment—that is to say, preventive maintenance that keeps the problem from developing in the first place. As Dr. Neil Baum, director of the New Orleans Impotence Foundation, says, "Men with poorly controlled diabetes have decreased sex drive as well as problems with impotence. Good control is associated with improvement in potency, libido, and sense of well-being."

FOR WOMEN:
Will my diabetes cause sexual problems?

Previously it had been thought that diabetes had little or no effect on either a woman's sexual performance or satisfaction. Even now, based on what diabetic women report to their doctors, it would seem that they reach a sexual climax just as often as nondiabetic women.

Still there are rumblings from some diabetes therapists—especially female diabetes therapists—that sex problems associated with diabetes are as common among women as among men. It's just that the male sex problems have been given more attention. This is not necessarily due to sexism. It may be due to the fact that sexual response is easier to measure with men than with women. (And easier for women to fake than men.)

The majority of women's sexual problems appear to be related to poor diabetes control. A woman understandably loses interest in sex when she is excessively tired and run down from being out of control. High blood sugar and the resulting sugar in the urine increase susceptibility to vaginal infections that cause swelling, itching, burning, and pain, which are hardly conducive to enthusiasm for sexual intercourse. These infections can be treated with salves (Monistat), but the only real cure is keeping your diabetes under control.

If a long-term diabetic woman develops neuropathy (damaged nerve cells)—again often as a result of poor control—it may involve the nerve fibers that stimulate the genitalia so that arousal may not occur, making intercourse painful because lubricating fluids are not released. Arthur Krosnick, M.D., writing in *Diabetes Forecast,* recommends the use of water-soluble lubricants, such as K-Y Lubricating Jelly, for this condition. He also states that "estrogen deficiency responds to vaginal creams. These creams are available by prescription and do not affect diabetes control."

Emotional factors associated with diabetes—anxiety, fear, anger, and, especially, depression—can significantly decrease a woman's desire for sex, especially since these negative emotions often result in (or are a result of) poor diabetes control.

Dr. Lois Jovanovic-Peterson, writing in *The Diabetic Woman,* neatly sums up the situation: "The best way to be sexy and enjoy sex, therefore, is to be happy, healthy, fit, and in good control of your blood-glucose levels."

She also offers this handy hint for insulin-taking diabetic women when things are going well in the sex department: "If a woman thoroughly enjoys the sexual encounter, the sheer exercise of the experience may result in a severe hypoglycemic episode. Thus, a woman needs to be prepared. She should adjust her insulin downward in anticipation of the evening, or if the evening happens to be on the spur of the moment, she should compensate by eating something afterward." *Bon appétit!*

Should I become pregnant?

We assume from this question that you have already wrestled through the basic Everywoman life decision of whether to have children and have concluded that you want to, but you worry about the effect your diabetes will have on your baby and vice versa.

The first consideration is: do you have any diabetes complications such as retinopathy (diabetic eye damage), neuropathy (nerve damage), or poor kidney function? If so, you may have to postpone the idea of becoming pregnant, because pregnancy could worsen the condition. Oddly enough, it can go both ways. In the case of retinopathy, Dr. Jovanovic-Peterson told us that "of one hundred women with retinopathy, 50 percent have no change, 25 percent get better, and 25 percent get worse with pregnancy." It is for this reason that before entering into a pregnancy you need to consult with your diabetes specialist to make sure you have a normal hemoglobin A_1C, with your gynecologist, with an ophthalmologist, and with a urologist.

If all systems are go, you can be cheered by the news that your chances of having a healthy baby are exactly the same as a non-diabetic woman's. The one great warning is to establish normal blood sugar (a normal A_1C) *before* becoming pregnant. Otherwise, you're in trouble from the start.

We must also forewarn you that a diabetic woman's pregnancy means a great intensification of self-care. Blood sugar must be monitored on a meter between five and ten times a day. Blood-sugar level must be kept between 60 and 90 before meals and less than 140 after meals during the entire term of the pregnancy. This means excessive risk of hypoglycemia for Type I's. That's why the pregnancy is sometimes harder on the husband than the wife.

Cost is also an important factor. The major expenses are blood-sugar-testing supplies and fetal monitoring (amniocenteses, ultrasounds, fetal-echo checks, and fetal nonstress tests). Not to scare you, but the cost of fetal testing for a Type I friend of ours was $3,650 in 1987.

If your main concern involves the ethics of producing a child with the possibility of diabetic heredity, that's a decision only you can make. Fortunately, the pattern of inheritance of diabetes is now much clearer, and the picture looks brighter than it did just a few years ago. Children of Type I diabetics have only a 2 to 6 percent chance of also becoming diabetic. Non-insulin-dependent diabetes is more inheritable. The children of Type II's have a 15 to 25 percent chance of becoming diabetic.

What is the best contraceptive for a woman to use?

Birth control for diabetic women is essentially the same as for non-diabetic women. The choice is up to the woman, her partner, and her gynecologist. The most commonly used method is the low-dose pill. These pills are not considered dangerous unless you have high blood pressure or retinopathy. Ordinarily they do not have an impact on your insulin doses, but in higher dosages they can change insulin requirements and thus it's best to keep in touch with your diabetes doctor and gynecologist about this.

The long-standing barrier methods are okay, also—diaphragms, condoms, and cervical sponges. For women who are certain they don't want to become pregnant in the future, sterilization (obviously) is the most reliable method.

One diabetic woman we talked to said she thinks the safest and most reliable method of contraception is a husband with a vasectomy.

And, finally, our editor, who feels we should present every possible option in this book, offers the reminder, "There's always celibacy."

Can people with diabetes travel?

Anyone who knows the two of us at all will realize that we would consider that question as ridiculous as asking "Can people with diabetes breathe?" Travel is that much a part of our lives—and we feel it should be that much a part of yours.

On this shrinking planet, your job may require you to travel all over the country or even all over dozens of other countries. Never let your diabetes stop you. If you keep yourself under good control and plan ahead, you'll make business trips with as much ease and success as the nondiabetic next person. As a matter of fact, because of your good health habits, you may well be brighter and more alert and ready for the work than nondiabetics, who may feel a little headachy from airline cocktails or drowsy from carousing.

Terrence Mason, a trainer for the Grantmanship Center in Los Angeles, spends an estimated 60 to 70 percent of his time traveling all over the world. In the Summer 1989 issue of *Living Well with Diabetes,* the quarterly journal published by the International Diabetes Center in Minneapolis, Minnesota, Mason says that because he is black he has to recognize that he may encounter prejudices and stereotyping in his travels and be prepared for them. Once when he needed to purchase syringes he found that because of his color he was automatically suspected of being a drug user. "I could go into places, as middle-class and as old as I am," he says, "and there'd be many places that just wouldn't sell me syringes." His doctor later explained that he could always go to a hospital emergency room and get syringes. But now he also carries his doctor's phone number so he can call to request that a prescription be prepared by another doctor in the city where he's traveling. That's a good idea for anyone of any color.

Carrying a letter from your doctor explaining that you have diabetes and outlining your treatment needs is also a good idea. This is not just to help you get syringes or insulin or whatever else you need in an emergency, but to identify you as a diabetic in case customs inspectors notice your syringes. This is especially true for young people; we know of one young woman on a school-sponsored educational tour who was interrogated by the authorities at one border because of her syringes. They wound up believing her, but it was a very disturbing experience for her because the whole tour group was held up while she was being worked over. It was an experience that could have been avoided with a doctor's letter and plenty of diabetes identification.

In the back of our book *The Peripatetic Diabetic,* we include identification information for insulin-taking diabetics in Danish, Dutch, Finnish, French, German, Greek, Italian, Japanese, Norwegian, Portuguese, Russian, Spanish, and Swedish. Feel free to copy any of those you might need. If you can't locate the book, write to us at Prana Publications (See Recommended Reading; Magazines, *Diabetic Reader*) and tell us which ID you need; we'll be glad to run off a copy and send it to you.

Even more important than business travel, though, is the travel you do for pleasure and mind expansion. To our way of thinking, the vacation spent puttering around the house is not a vacation at all. A true vacation gets you away from home and away from the routine demands on your time and the routine worries that constantly nibble on your subconscious.

The strange thing is that if you just get away for a short time— even a weekend—you feel so restored and unstressed that it's as if you'd had a month-long holiday.

If you're nervous about handling your diabetes away from home, you might try our "expanding circle" method of travel. Make your first trip a weekend jaunt to a very nearby town or, if you live in a large city, to another part of the same city. You can pretend you're on the opposite side of the earth, but you know you can get home fast or get in touch with your doctor if there's an emergency.

When you've proved to yourself that staying in a hotel and eating all your meals out poses no problems to you or your diabetes, expand the circle farther by going someplace about five hundred miles away. Next travel all the way across the country to a place you've always wanted to visit. Then try Canada or Hawaii—both have a foreign feeling and yet pose no language or food problems.

Finally, after you've had success in these areas, go to Europe or Asia or Australia or Africa or even Antarctica, if that's your pleasure. For the truth is that a diabetic can travel anywhere that diabetics live, and, of course, that's every country on earth.

Now that you're all hyped up and ready to go, here are a few of our favorite travel tips and precautions.

- Take double quantities of all diabetes and other medical supplies that you use. It may not be easy to find them, especially overseas, and besides, who wants to spend vacation time shopping in pharmacies? If you're a belt-and-suspenders type, as June is, carry half your supplies in one place and half in another so that if you should lose a purse or piece of luggage, you'll still be covered. Then, just to be on the absolutely safe side, carry along a prescription for any medication you take. Have your doctor make this for the generic name of the drug, since the trade name may vary from country to country.

- Try to go to just one place. In the United States make it one city or national park or resort area; overseas, just one country. (A few years ago we actually went just to Rome for three weeks.) If you don't try to gulp down the whole world on a single vacation, you'll spend more time being there rather than going to a lot of different theres. You'll have more time on your feet exploring or playing than on your seat in a car or bus or train or plane. Your diabetes will show its appreciation. And if you go to only one country, you'll be able to do research ahead of time into the native cuisine to make your meals easier to figure, and more fun as well. You'll also be able to learn a few appropriate phrases in the language ("I am a diabetic." "Where is the restroom?" "Quick! Get me some sugar!").

- Sports vacations are wonderful. Not only do you get healthful and restoring exercise while you're there, but you can also take lessons to acquire (or hone) a skill like tennis or golf or skiing that will enrich you and make your whole life healthier.

- Two short vacations are better than one long one. You get the welcome release of a holiday at two different times of the year instead of just one. And it's true that it becomes wearisome to stay away from home for too long. June prefers vacations of one or two weeks, but if she's going overseas, she's willing to stretch it to three. Her basic rule: "I come home when all my clothes are dirty."

■ Take along two pairs of broken-in (*not* broken-down) shoes. If possible, change your shoes in the middle of the day. This helps prevent blisters. Walk and walk and walk and walk. You'll see more and get to *eat* more that way.

■ As you start your trip, make it a point to slip into what Olympic gold-medal marathon runner and attorney Frank Shorter calls his "travel mode." This means keeping relaxed and making a conscious effort not to let anything bother you. If there's a flight delay, no matter. If a crying baby is seated nearby, no matter. If someone whaps your ear with a flight bag when putting it in the overhead compartment, no matter. Remain in a semimeditative state, a kind of "serene mellowness," as Shorter puts it. Getting angry and upset over the inevitable annoyances associated with travel only hurts (and raises the blood sugar of) one person: you.

■ Another Shorter travel tip is to be especially pleasant to any of the service people you deal with on a trip. He finds that courtesy is usually returned in kind and often serves to iron out potential wrinkles in your trip (and on your brow).

■ Take all the normal precautions any prudent traveler—diabetic or not—would take. For example, be sure all your basic shots are up to date. Tetanus is a particularly important one because, in case of an accident, getting a tetanus shot on top of whatever other trauma you're experiencing just exacerbates the condition. If there's a flu going around, it usually goes around everywhere, so have a shot for that unless you've had one recently. You should check with your travel agent to see what extra shots are recommended for the places you're visiting and take those as well. Any shots you take should be taken well ahead of time. If you get a reaction to any of them, you don't want it to take place on the trip. Besides, it sometimes takes a while for the immunity to set in and keep you covered. Check to find out if your health insurance covers you in foreign countries; if it doesn't, talk to your travel or insurance agent about a special short-term policy to cover you while you're traveling.

■ For foreign travel, write to the International Diabetes Federation, International Association Center, 40 Washington St., 1050 Brussels, Belgium; phone 32-2-647-41-14 for a list of diabetes specialists. You might also purchase membership in the International Association for Medical Assistance to Travelers (IAMAT) for a 72-page directory of English-speaking doctors around the world. IAMAT's address: 417 Center St., Lewiston, NY 14092; phone 716-754-4883.

■ Two other handy things to take with you on a trip: a small but bright-beamed flashlight so you won't stub your toe while stumbling around strange hotel rooms in the dark looking for the bathroom or your testing materials or snacks or whatever you might need during the night for your diabetes care (this will also come in handy for reading menus in dark restaurants); and a friend or relative who understands diabetes and can help you cope with the unexpected.

■ Relax and have a good time.

Follow these rules and, indeed, the longest and most grueling of flights or bus, train, or car trips will seem shorter.

How can I get special diabetic meals on airplanes?

You can request them when you buy your tickets and the agent relays your order to the airline. If you later change your flight, you must inform the airline so that it can switch your meal order, too.

Virtually all airlines offer special diabetic trays. Once, however, when we flew United Airlines to Hawaii, the dietary-meal request slip was accidentally left on the tray. This showed that the same meal was being delivered to all those who had made these special requests for meals: diabetic, Hindu, Moslem, hypoglycemic, low calorie, low carbohydrate, low cholesterol, low fat, and low sodium. Clearly, a meal that tries to be appropriate for all of the above is not going to be totally right for any of them. And it wasn't. There was not a starch exchange to be found on the tray.

After years of trying on dozens of airlines, we've finally given up and now just take what comes. June can sort through it and pick out what she needs. After all, when immobilized on an airplane, a diabetic can eat very little anyway. It's better to concentrate not on food but rather on drinking lots of water (so you won't get dehydrated from the dry air in the cabin) and walking up and down the aisle as often as you can to keep your circulation chugging along. Drinking alcohol on a flight isn't too smart, either, since it, too, is dehydrating.

Naturally, you should bring along lots of snacks in case for some reason no food of any kind appears, or appears much later than you need it.

How can I avoid getting diarrhea when I travel in foreign countries?

Sometimes you can't. Each country has its own varieties of bacteria in the water and food. The very fact that these are different from the ones you're accustomed to causes the classic tourist problem.

Both Type I's and Type II's should, of course, do everything possible to protect themselves from diarrhea. In south-of-the-border countries where *turista* is a special threat, or overseas in less developed countries, drink only bottled water and avoid drinks containing ice. According to Maury Rosenbaum, who publishes the newsletter *The Diabetic Traveler* (P.O. Box 8223 RW, Stamford, CT 06905), ice actually preserves germs. He also advises always ordering carbonated water ("with gas") as carbonation adds acid and acidity kills microorganisms.

Brush your teeth using either bottled water or water you've boiled. Beware of carafes of water left on your dresser. They may well have been filled from the tap.

When all preventive measures fail, you should take some kind of antidiarrhea remedy. You'll need to consult your own doctor on this, but Dr. Peter Lodewick, writing in *The Diabetic Man*, recommends Lomotil and Imodium for diarrhea and Pepto-Bismol for nausea and cramping.

Besides taking a remedy for diarrhea, try to drink a cup of broth every hour and have bananas as your fruit exchange. This restores vital salts and potassium that are lost from your system in bouts of diarrhea. An effective folk remedy is camomile tea, known in Spanish as *té de manzanilla.*

Is it all right for me to have my ears pierced? Wear acrylic nails? Have a face-lift?

It seemed to be a good idea to group all these appearance-enhancing questions together since they have basically the same answer.

We first became aware of the ear-piercing problem when Barbara had hers pierced. She was made to sign a consent slip stating that she didn't have diabetes. Since she isn't diabetic, signing it posed no problem, but it did set her to thinking that it didn't seem fair to keep diabetics from getting their ears pierced if they wanted to. We checked with some of our experts.

Richard K. Bernstein, diabetic diabetologist of Mamaroneck, New York, was of the opinion that the restriction made sense because the vast majority of diabetics are in such poor control that it would be an infection risk for them.

Diana Guthrie, a diabetes nurse specialist, had a more positive approach: "So long as your blood sugars are normalized or near normalized, there should be no hesitation whatsoever in getting your ears pierced if the proper precautions that are taken for everybody else are taken for you."

Assuming you take care of this risk factor, you're left with only the dilemma of whether to sign the paper saying that you're *not* diabetic. Since the ear-piercing brigade is probably having you sign only to protect itself in the event of an infection, it would seem that all you're doing is denying yourself legal recourse if something should go wrong. But whether to sign is a moral question rather than a diabetic one, and we aren't the best source of the answer.

The reason we brought up the question of acrylic nails is that we know diabetics are more susceptible to nail fungus than others. Attaching these nails might therefore cause fungus to develop or spread. Diana Guthrie again set our minds at ease. She explains: "Glued-on nails do not enhance the development of fungal infections so long as careful hand-washing techniques are routinely instituted and the fungal organism is not overwhelmingly present." One of our former SugarFree employees, Melanie Epperson, who had her own nail business, echoed this sentiment. She had several diabetic clients who had acrylic nails, and not one had ever had a problem with them.

And now we get to the biggie—a face-lift. We won't debate here the advisability of cosmetic surgery (which is questionable unless the surgery is done to correct something like a cleft palate or to repair the ravages of an accident). If you do decide, for whatever personal reasons, that you would like to have a face-lift, the question is, Should your diabetes stand in your way? Again we hear good news from Diana Guthrie: "The advisability of anyone getting a face-lift or other cosmetic surgery is the same as for any surgical procedure. If someone has diabetes and it is *under control,* they probably will heal faster and better than even the nondiabetic. There should be no hesitation to do surgical procedures, so long as the service of a knowledgeable physician is available to manage the diabetes before, during, and after the procedure." Lois Jovanovic-Peterson agrees. This goes along with her philosophy that diabetics who are in control can do virtually anything they'd do if they weren't diabetic.

So the answer to all of the above (and all of life) is yes, if your diabetes is *under control.*

Is it all right to use generic drugs?

Before we answer that, we'd like you to have an understanding of what generic drugs are. We'd long been confused about them ourselves, so we asked Mike Voelker, Pharm. D., Manager, National Medical Care in Chatsworth, California, to explain them. The first thing we found out surprised us: pharmacies actually make a greater percentage of profit on generics than on brand names, so if your pharmacist discourages you from purchasing a certain generic, he's doing it for professional reasons and not out of some sordid profit motive.

Mike further explains that generic drugs (drugs not protected by trademark) are in demand today for many valid reasons. First, insurance companies and other health-cost payment systems are encouraging their members to use generic drugs by offering people a lower copayment if they do. Second, the FDA is shortening the time period for trade-name drugs to become generic. And third, over the next three to four years, if the federal government (Medicare) phases in payments for prescription drugs (just as the state of California now does with its Medi-Cal drug program), it will probably demand that generic medications be provided whenever possible.

For the above reasons, it's safe to say that generics are here to stay. But . . . buyer, beware! Some warnings are in order. Brand-name drugs and their generic forms are not necessarily identical. Switching to a generic without proper precautions may cause serious problems. To understand the possible difficulties, you have to understand what generic drugs are and how they're made.

A generic drug has exactly the same amount of the active ingredient as the trade-name product. The active ingredient by weight, however, makes up only a fraction of the total weight of the tablet or capsule. For example, a Lanoxin 0.25 mg tablet weighs about 1.5 mg, but the active ingredient (Digoxin) makes up only about 10 percent of the total weight of the tablet. The other 90 percent comprises what pharmacists call excipients—fillers, binding agents, coloring, etc. It is these extra ingredients that very often determine how much of the active drug is absorbed into the bloodstream and how quickly. In some cases more drug is absorbed and in other cases less. This difference can be critical, depending on the type of drug you're using.

With the following classes of drugs, you and your doctor and pharmacist must be extremely careful when changing to the generic form:

- cardiovascular drugs (Digoxin, Inderal, etc.)
- hormone and related drugs (Premarin)

- psychotherapeutic drugs (Thorazine, Elavil, etc.)
- anticonvulsants (Dilantin)
- oral hypoglycemics (Orinase, Diabenese, etc.)

A diabetic, for example, can switch from the trade name Orinase to the generic tolbutamide, but you should always ask your physician first. When the switch is made, you must be very diligent about testing for hyper- or hypoglycemia so you can determine whether the generic is being absorbed in the same way as the trade-name pill. Then, once you have successfully switched, you have to make sure you are always provided with that particular brand of generic, because *generics also differ from brand to brand.* This is another complication, which means that only those in the know can protect themselves from drug overdose or underdose.

With classes of drugs not on the above list, such as antibiotics and analgesics, it is perfectly okay to switch to a generic brand without any special monitoring.

The final word on generics, then, is to go ahead and enjoy the savings they offer, but make sure that you, your physician, and your pharmacist work as a team to ensure their safe and efficacious use.

For People with Type I (Insulin-Dependent) Diabetes

. . . .

Being on insulin is like being involved in a passionate yet turbulent marriage, one of those "can't live with; can't live without" situations.

In the case of your relationship with your insulin there are times—especially after a particularly devastating or embarrassing insulin reaction—that you feel you can't possibly live with it, no, not one minute longer. But you have no choice. You and insulin are partners, locked together inextricably forever. No divorce allowed.

Admittedly, insulin is a difficult and demanding helpmate. There's the needle and the several-times-a-day injections; the constant lookout for insulin shock; the need to have something sugary available at all times; the problem of keeping medical supplies in stock; the precise food requirements, with eating too little as big a mistake as eating too much; the necessity of stuffing some therapeutic food down for insulin's sake when you're not even hungry, the inevitable snacks between meals and at bedtime, and the inability of family, friends, and co-workers to comprehend what's going on in your rocky relationship with insulin. Then there's the expense of your marriage to insulin. No one ever had a more incorrigible spendthrift of a spouse. Living with insulin uses up big dollars that you'd rather spend on pleasures—and even sometimes need to spend on necessities.

And yet despite everything you must love your insulin. It gives you the most precious gift of all: the gift of life itself. Before its discovery in 1921, you'd have been a goner. While it's not a cure for diabetes, as some people erroneously think it is, it's the next-best thing; in fact the *only* thing there is.

So since you're stuck (!) with insulin until they find that fabled cure that's always "just ten years away," you have to make the best of it. To help you do that, we'll now give you some insulin marital counseling in the hope that you will learn to live with your insulin happily—or at least with respect and understanding—ever after and that you will celebrate your golden and even your diamond anniversary together.

What is insulin?

Insulin, as we mentioned earlier, is the hormone that helps the body cells take up sugar from the blood. As a Type I diabetic, you must inject insulin to replace your body's lack of the hormone. The amount to be injected every day depends on whether your body is producing none or only a small amount. If it is producing none, your injections are a substitute for your own insulin; if it is producing some, you have to augment your own insulin with injections. Your physician will determine how much insulin you need and which kinds.

There are two kinds of insulin: fast-acting and slow-acting. Fast-acting insulin is called Regular insulin or Semi-lente. It begins acting in about half an hour and lasts approximately one to five hours. The slow-acting insulins are divided into two types: intermediate-acting and long-acting. Intermediate-acting insulins are called NPH and Lente. These begin acting in about an hour and a half and last approximately twelve to twenty-four hours. Ultralente is the only long-acting insulin. It begins to take effect in one to three hours and can last up to thirty-six hours. Most diabetics take a combination of fast-acting and intermediate- or long-acting insulins.

Injectable insulins come in bottles of ten cubic centimeters each. Fast-acting insulin is clear, and slow-acting is cloudy. Insulin is measured in units. All insulin sold in the United States is of the same concentration: U100, which means that there are one hundred units of insulin in each cubic centimeter. So a ten-cubic centimeter bottle would contain one thousand units of insulin. If your dosage of insulin is ten units a day, then a bottle of insulin will contain 100 doses.

The insulins sold in the United States are manufactured by two major companies: Eli Lilly and Novo Nordisk. All insulin used to be made from the pancreas of pigs and steers. Though many people still use animal insulin, the new human insulins made in laboratories by DNA technology are preferred. Since this synthetic human insulin is identical to the body's own, it does not cause antibodies or allergic reactions, and is absorbed more quickly. Human insulins are extremely pure (99.999 percent) compared with the animal insulins of the past. And even the newer animal insulins called "purified" are 99.99 percent pure. So if you must take insulin, at least you know that it is of unimpeachable quality.

Most physicians think everyone should now use human insulin. Oddly enough, though, not all old-time diabetics can successfully switch to human insulin and maintain the same control they had with animal insulin. There are also diabetics who cannot afford to change from the old beef-pork combination because it is much less expensive than human or purified pork. (We hope that's not you.)

Insulins now have such great variety that you must make absolutely certain when you go shopping that you're getting exactly what your doctor prescribed and even the same brand he prescribed. Take the empty bottle with you. Another tip: keep a backup supply of at least one bottle, as not all pharmacies stock all varieties of insulin, and you may dash out to replace your vial only to find that your pharmacy has none.

Why can't I just take my insulin in a pill?

Insulin is a protein, and if it were delivered in pill form, the stomach would digest it the way it would a hamburger; you'd get no benefit from it. Researchers are now working on encapsulating insulin in a substance that would allow it to pass through the stomach without being digested and then be released in the intestine, but they have been working on it for a long time.

Since people don't like to have to inject insulin, many other possibilities have been and are still being looked into. These include insulin suppositories, nasal spray, and insulin patches. Insulin suppositories were developed in Israel, but were never distributed widely, probably because they would be no more popular than injections. Nasal spray has so far not been shown to absorb evenly. Insulin patches are being researched by Americare Transtech Incorporated. They allow insulin to be absorbed through the skin. If the research is successful and the FDA approves the technology, then a company has to be found to manufacture the patches.

Once you start taking insulin, do you have to take it for the rest of your life?

If you're a Type I diabetic, yes, you're probably stuck (!) with it. Occasionally after children or young people are first diagnosed and start using insulin, there comes a honeymoon period. The disease seems to fade away, they can stop taking insulin, and their family believes a miracle has occurred and they are cured. Not so. Like all honeymoons, the diabetes honeymoon eventually comes to an end, and insulin injections must begin again. (But enjoy it while it lasts.)

Sometimes if you're a Type II you may be on insulin only until you get your weight down.

Also, diabetics who aren't normally on insulin may have to take it when they're sick or have an infection or are pregnant. When they're well again, or the baby is delivered, they can stop.

Where and how do I inject insulin?

Insulin can be injected into the arm, abdomen, buttocks, or thigh. To make sure you stay within the proper area of each of these sites, you can order the pamphlet *Site Selection and Rotation* from Becton

Dickinson Consumer Products, One Becton Drive, Franklin Lakes, NJ 07417-1883 (1-800-526-4650).

It's very important to rotate your injections within each area, because there are differences in the speed with which insulin is absorbed, depending on where it is injected. Injection in the abdomen is fastest—30 to 50 percent faster than in other areas; next fastest are arms and legs. The usual lag time for the abdomen is 30 to 40 minutes, while in the arm or leg the time lag is usually around 40 to 50 minutes. Insulin also acts faster in places that are lean rather than fat. According to Dr. Jay S. Skyler, professor of medicine, pediatrics, and psychology at the University of Miami School of Medicine, it is preferable to inject all before-meal shots of regular insulin into the abdomen for faster action. This will help prevent post-meal blood sugar from being too high.

How and when do I inject insulin?

Your doctor or nurse educator will teach you the injection technique and help you practice until you feel confident, though not necessarily as relaxed about it as you'd like to. The doctor will prescribe the type or types of insulin to use and the dosage.

Standard instructions have always been to take your insulin shot one half hour before eating. However, if you test your blood sugar before your meals—and you should!—it's preferable to use your test result as a guide to timing. The rationale behind this is that you can make adjustments in injection timing so the insulin's peak action will match the entry of glucose into your blood from the food you eat. Glucose starts arriving in your intestinal tract within ten minutes of eating, but insulin doesn't even begin to get going for over fifteen minutes. That's why the timing guidelines developed by Doctors David S. Schade, Mark R. Burge, and Patrick J. Boyle, of the University of New Mexico School of Medicine in Albuquerque, are so valuable. They suggest that you test your blood sugar forty-five minutes before the meal, then time your insulin injection according to your blood sugar level. These are the Schade/Burge/Boyle guidelines:

Blood Sugar 45 Minutes Prior to Meal	When to Take Your Insulin
50 mg/dl or less	after you finish the meal
50 to 70 mg/dl	just before starting the meal
70 to 120 mg/dl	15 minutes before the meal
120 to 180 mg/dl	30 minutes before the meal
Over 180 mg/dl	45 minutes before the meal

Adapted from an article in *Diabetes Forecast,* July 1993, with permission of the authors.

How can I get over my fear of the needle?

First of all, don't feel you're more cowardly than anyone else. We've never met any people who enjoyed sticking themselves with a needle. (And in fact, we'd rather not meet any.) We have met several, though, who swore they'd never be able to do it, but when the golden moment arrived they found they could, as Lady Macbeth put it, screw their courage to the sticking place.

Most insulin-dependent diabetics who inject themselves—and many do it two or three times a day for better management—get so used to it that it's fairly routine. (We won't give you the nonsense that "it becomes like brushing your teeth.")

Sometimes people can inject themselves for years without being bothered by it. Then suddenly they begin building up dread again. If you haven't yet conquered your fear or if you find it suddenly reappearing, here's what you can do about it.

- If you have the habit of worrying about the injection and how much it's going to hurt, instead picture yourself doing it easily and without pain. Positive thinking brings about positive results.

- If you've been having someone else give you shots, start giving them yourself. Not only is this necessary in case of emergencies, but you'll reinforce your feelings of competence. You may even discover that it hurts less when you do it yourself. We tend to tense our muscles when someone else is taking a poke at us.

- Relax. Those tense muscles we just mentioned not only make the shot hurt more but can also cause bruising. (And getting bruises is not a way to make yourself fear the needle less.)

- June found that when she switched from one to three shots a day, and then later on to five, an amazing change took place: she lost all dread of the needle. This may sound ridiculous, but it's true. Our explanation is that the more often you do it, the less time you'll have to build up a wall of worry. You inject your insulin as calmly as you'd do any other daily task.

A dividend you get from mastering your insulin injections is a feeling of power, an "If I can do this, I can do anything" feeling. You'll find you become a stronger person in every way.

Now, having given you this pep talk to make you positively panting with eagerness to stick yourself with a needle, we'll deliver the news that you don't have to if you don't want to. Modern technology strikes again to make diabetes self-care easier and less traumatic.

What is an automatic injector?

An automatic injector takes a loaded syringe and shoots it into you so quickly that you hardly know it happened. It gives you perfect injection technique, and since you don't even see the needle in the device, it does a lot toward keeping you relaxed. Not only do these devices eliminate the fear and pain, but can reach a lot of new injection territory and reach it with one hand—especially important for parents of small children, for whom the statement "This hurts me more than it does you" is often true. When a parent uses one of these devices, everybody is happier. People with arthritis or other dexterity problems also find these a boon. But the greatest advantage of automatic injectors is that they facilitate the multiple injections many people need to keep their diabetes under control and help them avoid complications.

The currently available injectors include the Injectomatic (Kendall-Futuro), the Autojector (Ulster Scientific), the Inject-Ease (Palco), and the Instaject II (Jordan Medical). Some are pictured below. The prices range between $20 and $50. Most injectors can accommodate all sizes and brands of syringes. (Note: The Injecto-matic is usable only with Monoject syringes, which isn't too surpris-ing since Kendall-Futuro makes both.)

After the injector zaps in the needle, you press the syringe plunger to release the insulin. (With the Autojector the insulin is re-leased automatically.)

Automatic Injectors

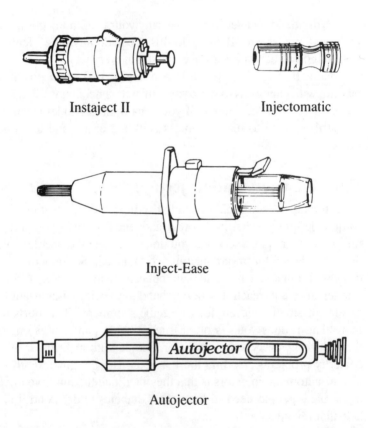

Instaject II   Injectomatic

Inject-Ease

Autojector

Even with an automatic injector, though, it's true you're still using a needle, and if needles are intrinsically horrifying to you, there is yet another alternative.

What is a jet injector?

Using a jet injector is the only way at present to take insulin without using a needle. (True, there are a few diabetic pioneers trying out some kind of implanted "artificial pancreas," but so far that is strictly experimental and a long way from everyday use.)

With a jet, the insulin itself becomes like a needle because it is shot in with such jetlike speed. All you feel is something like snapping your finger against your skin. You can mix insulins just as you can with needles. These instruments are way beyond the experimental stage, having been in use since 1979. June got her first jet in 1985 and has used three different models since. Over that period jets have been constantly improved technically, decreased in size, simplified, and gone down in price.

We feel that with the DCCT proving the benefits of multiple injections for tight control, the time has come for jets to be more widely prescribed and used. Many people would happily switch to tighter control if only they could do it without syringes and needles. If you suffer from true needle phobia, these needleless injectors are about the only answer for you.

But to our minds, escaping from needles is only a secondary reason for using a jet. Their greatest advantage, besides encouraging you to take more shots per day, is that they improve control, often with less insulin. When you inject with a needle, the insulin can pool at the injection site (this is called "depoting" in the trade), and the insulin is not absorbed as quickly as it should be, so it may not be there when you need it to cover a meal. Then, whammo, it's released later when you *don't* need it, and your blood sugar plummets. Jets disperse the insulin under the skin in a spray and that explains its quicker and more uniform absorption. When insulin's action is more predictable, you have more consistent control of your blood sugar.

Jet injectors do not, of course, give ideal injections for everybody. Some people can use them and love them while others have problems. Some can get pain-free, bruise-free injections in any injection location, while others can get good shots only in the abdomen, or only in the thighs, but then that's often true of syringes as well.

When the world of health care was more affluent, you could go to a diabetes center and have a jet demonstration and lesson and all the follow-up you needed to make the instrument work for you, but what with all the cutbacks such service is scarce now. Fortunately, though, most jet manufacturers have a thirty-day trial period. (In some cases there is a restocking fee if you decide to return it.) The instrument is sent to you via mail order and a video is supplied for instruction. The jet injector companies also have 800 numbers for help from an experienced customer service staff.

Jets require a doctor's prescription and a fairly large initial investment—between $500 and $700. Insurance coverage is fairly good and getting better, especially if you get pre-approval. The cost of the instrument is made up in about three years because of savings on syringe purchases and reduced insulin requirements.

The two most experienced manufacturers and the two whose instruments June is familiar with are Medi-Ject Corporation, 1840 Berkshire Lane, Minneapolis, MN 55441 (1-800-328-3074). (Three models, around $795 each); Vitajet Corporation, 27075 Cabot Rd. #102, Laguna Hills, CA 92653 (1-800-848-2538). (Two models, around $675 each.)

These companies are constantly working on improvements in their instruments, trying to produce more user-friendly and less costly versions. Here are illustrations of two of the current models.

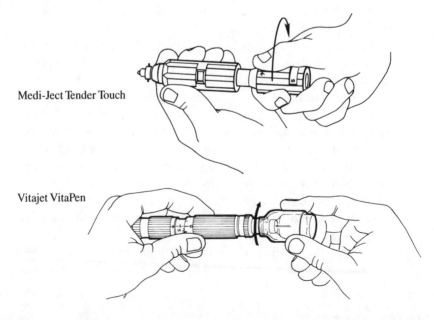

Medi-Ject Tender Touch

Vitajet VitaPen

Is the insulin-infusion pump I've heard about another way of getting off needles?

Not exactly, but it *is* a way to achieve the best possible control. That is why 59 percent of the intensive group in the DCCT were on pump therapy at least part of the time, and most of them chose to stay on it when the study ended, if they could afford to when they had to pay the costs themselves (see table on page 101).

Dr. Alan O. Marcus, writing in *Practical Diabetology* (November 1992), defined those people who are the best prospects for pump therapy, or as the physicians call it, "continuous subcutaneous insulin infusion." You are a good candidate if (1) you desire life-style flexibility, (2) you have unacceptable diabetes control, (3) you have chronic complications of diabetes, or (4) you want to become pregnant. The strongest candidates are those whose lifestyle is "active and variable." Physicians always stress that to be successful on a pump you must be highly motivated to use one, because pumps are not an *easier* way to good control, but a *better* way.

Pumps have been in use for fifteen years and have become highly sophisticated marvels of technology. They are now compact and sturdy, weigh only a little over three ounces, are battery operated, and highly programmable.

You wear the pump on a belt or strapped to your leg or anywhere it's convenient. At specific intervals the pump delivers regular insulin only. Regular insulin acts consistently, unlike intermediate and long-acting insulins, which have unpredictable absorption. The insulin travels through a slender, flexible tube and enters your body via a needle or, better still, a cannula (a tiny plastic tube) that is inserted under your skin at any normal injection site, usually the abdominal area. The needle or cannula stays in place for one to three days and then is rotated to a different spot, just as you change injection sites when using syringes and needles.

When it's time for a meal, you press a button to release the appropriate amount of regular insulin to cover the meal. Most pump wearers figure their mealtime insulin needs by testing their blood sugar and then counting the grams of carbohydrates they're going to eat.

One of the most valuable features of modern pumps is their

programmability. For example, people who inject long-acting insulin often get low blood sugar in the middle of the night and then
their blood sugar goes up in the very early morning (a condition
known as the dawn phenomenon). The pump wearer can program
the pump to deliver less insulin during the period when blood sugar
is likely to be down and more insulin for the dawn blood-sugar rise.

You have to work very closely with your diabetes health-care
team during the period when you're finding out what your body's
metabolic requirements are for insulin, the daily fluctuations of
your blood sugar, and how insulin sensitive or insulin resistant you
are in order to discover how much insulin will cover how many
grams of carbohydrate for you. But after all that's worked out, you
can have amazing control and amazing flexibility in your lifestyle
and mealtimes.

The best way for you to understand what pump wearing is like
is to hear it from pump wearers themselves. First, here's Pat Ockel
of San Diego:

> I got my MiniMed just before I went on an African safari in June
> 1987. It was one of the smallest pumps available at that time and it
> could get wet without being harmed; it had the largest reservoir (it
> carried 300 units of insulin); and it worked off three small batteries
> that could be found at most drugstores, even in Africa.
>
> After I got my MiniMed pump, my husband said that my
> moods really smoothed out compared to when I was on shots. Also, I
> haven't had any bad reactions the way I used to with syringes. The
> strange thing is that, since I use a Sof-set instead of having a needle
> inserted all the time, I'm not actually aware that it's there. And it cer-
> tainly makes it convenient for eating at restaurants when you just pull
> the pump out and take your dose right at the table.

And now here's Tom Chuchvara of Van Nuys, California:

> I had been on insulin injections for nine years when low blood sugars
> became frequent, unpredictable and at times life-threatening. I tested
> ten to twelve times a day and sometimes in the middle of the night to
> catch them before they happened, but I could not predict them.
>
> I was sure the lows were due to my physically active life-style of

drumming, surfing, running and weightlifting. I finally decided that a choice had to be made: either reduce the physical activity or find a program compatible with it. That's when I discovered the Disetronic H-Tron V100 insulin pump. This pump provides a feature that allows the user to adjust the rate at which insulin is pumped in order to match the level of physical activity at any given time.

The Disetronic has been part of my new program for over a year now. It allows me to manage my diabetes in accordance with my diet and the type of physical activity I choose, including surfing. My diabetes management has improved tremendously and I am now under good control. High and low blood sugars are extremely rare, and I am free to live as I want to.

For further information on pumps, write or call Disetronic Medical Systems, Inc., 13005 16th Avenue North, Suite 500, Plymouth, MN 55441 (1-800-688-4578), or MiniMed Technologies, Inc., 12744 San Fernando Rd., Sylmar, CA 91342 (1-800-933-3322).

What if I forget to take my insulin injection?

At least you'll know you're not obsessed with your disease. But if this happens more than once in a great while, you'll need to devise some kind of reminder system, like a nagging husband, wife, or parent. If you have small children, you can give them a penny each time you take the shot. (They'll never forget, but don't let them con you into taking your shot twice.) When it does dawn on you that you forgot your shot, take your blood sugar and see what's happening. Call your doctor, who can probably help you decide how much insulin to take, if any. Much depends on what kind of insulin you take and how many shots a day you take, so general advice is of no help.

Sometimes the problem is even worse. It's remembering whether or not you took the insulin. Then you have to worry about getting a double dose or no dose at all. If you use disposable needles (doesn't everyone?), you can look into the wastebasket and find out. If you're at a total loss and can't figure out whether you did or didn't, the safer course is not to take a shot. Think how tough it would be and how much time it would take to eat all the extra food the double injection would require, not to mention the weight it would put on. There's no doubt that a good memory is a help to a diabetic.

When I'm sick and can't eat, do I stop taking insulin?

That's a good question, as politicians being interviewed by reporters like to say. The answer is no, no, a thousand times no. If you have severe nausea and vomiting and can't keep anything down, you can sometimes reduce your normal daily insulin dose by one-half or two-thirds (if your blood sugars are normal). But more often when you're sick, your blood sugar goes up and you need more insulin, not less. (Illness makes insulin less effective.) Sometimes your doctor (keep in touch when you're sick) will prescribe additional shots of regular (fast-acting) insulin before each meal.

For sick days when you can't eat solid food, the usual recommendation is to sip ginger ale (to control nausea and to satisfy your insulin) and to drink clear broth or fruit juices every hour.

Whenever you're sick, especially with the flu, a cold, an injury, or an infection, you have to watch your diabetes more closely. Take your blood sugar every few hours. If it's over 240, check your urine for ketones. If ketones appear, call your doctor immediately. Blood-sugar levels can go very high during illness, and your doctor can help you bring them down safely. But don't just sit there—or lie there—and do nothing. This is not a situation you can safely ignore.

Do insulin syringes and needles require a prescription?

This one's a real puzzler. The answer is that they do and they don't. In California, for example, most pharmacists require only the diabetic's signature, not the doctor's. Some states, however, insist on a doctor's prescription. The laws vary from state to state, and the interpretation of the laws varies from pharmacy to pharmacy.

We've never tried purchasing this equipment out of state or overseas, but June always carries a doctor's prescription in case the occasion should ever arise.

Do I need to clean the skin with alcohol before I inject?

We hate to advocate unhygienic practices, but we also hate for you to get all agitated and upset if you don't have any alcohol or an alcohol swab along when you need to take a shot.

For what it's worth, June never cleans the injection site with alcohol—unless, of course, she hasn't been able to bathe on a daily basis. One doctor told us there was a British study in which they gave five thousand injections using alcohol and five thousand without. There were only five infections in the whole lot, and all those were in cases where alcohol had been used! (The doctor laughed and said maybe the alcohol irritated the bacteria and stirred them into action.)

How do I take care of my bottles of insulin?

Bottles is the correct word, because you should have more than one on hand. The backup supply should be kept in the refrigerator (not in the coldest part, where it might freeze, and certainly not in the freezer compartment). The vial you're using (or vials, if you use more than one kind) can stay at room temperature, providing it is not over 86 degrees. Insulin manufacturers usually recommend refrigeration between shots, but cold insulin causes more pain when injected and does not absorb as well. Insulin remains stable for one month without refrigeration. Always write the date you opened it on the bottle and discard it after a month.

You should, by the way, always watch the expiration date on your insulin. If you use it after that date, it may not be as effective. For that reason, you can't stock up on huge quantities of insulin when you find it on sale. That's not a good idea anyway, as you might change insulins.

When you find yourself out of control, the first thing to do is check the date on the insulin you're using. If it's slightly out-of-date or has been open over a month, throw it away. (It usually turns out that the insulin was not at fault.)

It's perfectly okay to carry your insulin in your purse or pocket (in a protective case of some kind) when you're not going to be taking your injection at home. Insulin is pretty hardy stuff. You just have to be careful not to freeze it or expose it to high temperatures (above one hundred degrees Fahrenheit).

When traveling you don't have to worry about keeping your insulin refrigerated, but you do have to worry about where to keep it. In airplanes, don't put your insulin in the luggage you check. Keep it in your pocket, purse, or hand luggage, both because the cargo hold may be too cold and because your luggage may get lost along the way. If you're traveling by automobile, don't leave your insulin in a closed car in the hot sun because the temperature can rise to damaging heights.

Many people like to buy an insulated carrying case for insulin, especially if they're planning a trip to an extremely hot or cold climate. The safest container, which works both ways, is also unfortunately the largest. It's the Medicool, which has a prerefrigeratable section that will keep insulin cool even in a hundred-degree oven. Unrefrigerated, the same section keeps insulin from freezing. The Dia-Pod also does double duty. It is an ultralight holder made of the tiniest of foam beads for maximum insulation. And the Insul-Tote is a foam-insulated bag that includes a refreezable refrigerant. New kinds of cases are constantly appearing, so watch for the one that suits you. These sorts of products can be purchased at most diabetes supply centers.

What causes those lumps that I sometimes get after a shot?

It could be that you've injected too frequently in the same place or that you're allergic to the kind of insulin you're using—or both. Try to be more conscientious about rotating the injection site. If the lumps continue to appear, tell your doctor, who may change the type of insulin you're using.

Some people get skin indentations or depressions instead of lumps. These are caused by losing fat wherever you inject insulin (fat atrophy). The correction for both problems, if you aren't on human insulin now, is often to change to human.

Can I get along on one shot of intermediate-acting insulin a day?

Almost definitely not. The therapeutic life of human NPH (the length of time it controls blood sugar) is only twelve to fourteen hours. The other intermediate-acting insulin, Lente, controls for only fourteen to sixteen hours. You can see that using only one shot of either of these insulins would leave you uncovered for a lot of time during a twenty-four-hour period. Not only that, but taking it in one shot would mean that the insulin would peak once, possibly at a time when you very likely wouldn't have planned to have your main meal. You'd have to feed your insulin when it demanded it and then not be able to eat when you (and everyone else) wanted to. So not only is one shot bad therapy, it makes for a rigid and unpleasant life.

Dr. Lois Jovanovic-Peterson does admit that people who still have some pancreatic function, mostly Type II's, can get along on only one shot of NPH. If you always have normal fasting blood sugars on the one-shot-a-day plan, you are among the few lucky ones who can do it. Dr. Jovanovic-Peterson emphasizes, though, that the vast majority of Type I diabetics who have no pancreatic function can't possibly have good control with one shot of NPH a day—no matter how much they'd love to do it.

You keep talking about taking all those injections to keep blood sugar normal. How do I handle it when I'm out at restaurants?

It's not all that difficult, thanks to the many helpful devices the diabeticization of America has produced.

You can load your syringe at home and carry it in a PDI (pre-drawn insulin) case, which was invented by a diabetic who needed it himself. The case is slim and unobtrusive, yet it's large enough to hold two predrawn syringes. In the restaurant restroom or even in the car prior to entering the restaurant, it's quick and easy to take your shot even if the lighting isn't bright enough for measuring your insulin.

Another new development that's particularly handy for inject-ing away from home is the NovolinPen. You load it with a cartridge of Novolin regular, NPH, or 70/30 (70 percent NPH, 30 percent reg-ular). Each cartridge contains 150 units of insulin. You can dial in the number of units you want to take (from 2 to 36 in 2-unit incre-ments) and shoot it in. You change the disposable needle at the end of the pen as needed.

The latest thing for people who take 70/30 insulin is the Novolin 70/30 Prefilled, a disposable syringe prefilled with 150 units of Novolin 70/30 human insulin. You use it with the dispos-able needles of the NovolinPen. It lasts from three to five days, de-pending on your dosage.

How do I adjust my insulin when I fly and change time zones?

That depends strictly on your insulin schedule, what kind of insulin you take, and how many shots a day you require. And there's more than one method for calculating the adjustments.

To give you a basic understanding of the problem, remember that time change occurs only when you fly east or west, not north or south. Flying from west to east, your day is shortened. Flying from east to west, it is lengthened. So when flying east, you lower your dosage; when flying west, you increase it. *But* if the change is not more than four hours, you don't need to take any special action. Likewise, if your total insulin dose is small—only ten or fifteen units—you can probably get by without any change.

If you monitor your blood sugar frequently, you can stay out of trouble and in control, no matter what. Knowing how to adjust in-sulin according to blood sugar and giving yourself supplements of regular insulin makes the whole thing easy. Otherwise, discuss your insulin program with your physician or nurse educator. First prepare yourself if you can by reading about the different ways to handle the situation. Read *The Joslin Diabetes Manual* or *Controlling Diabetes the Easy Way* by Stanley Mirsky (see Recommended Reading) or any other basic diabetes-education book that covers the subject.

Airborne-injection tip: When you take an insulin injection in a plane, do not inject air into the bottle. If you do, because of the difference in air pressure the plunger will fight you and make it difficult to measure accurately.

Is it all right to have low blood sugar?

No. Low blood sugar—or insulin reaction, as low blood sugar is often called—can be very hazardous for a diabetic because you become irritable, befuddled, uncoordinated, and, in extreme cases, unconscious. Automobile accidents are not the only possible danger. One of our friends fell in his swimming pool when he blacked out during an insulin reaction and was lucky enough to be awakened by the water and make it to the side and climb out. Maybe you read the story of Candy Sangster, who became unconscious during a weekend at home alone. She was saved by her dog, Jet, who went outside and barked until the neighbors decided to dial 911. Jet, a six-year-old Doberman, was named the Ken-L-Ration Dog Hero of the Year in 1986 for his dramatic lifesaving exploit. So if you don't own a dog, don't be lax about hypoglycemia.

The most logical way to check to see if you're having an insulin reaction is to take your blood sugar. You should also learn to recognize the characteristic physical and/or mental changes that take place. The difficulty is not only that these are very diverse, individualized, and vary from occasion to occasion but that many people fail to notice them. Psychologist Daniel J. Cox, Ph.D., in a study published in *Diabetes Care* (February 1993) found that in his group only 50 percent of the lows were recognized. He also found out that the most frequently recognized symptoms were trembling, difficulty concentrating, confusion, and pounding heart. Notice that half of these are mental rather than physical.

A serious problem that has surfaced recently is one called "hypoglycemic unawareness" or more descriptively "hypoglycemia without warning." Robert S. Dinsmoor, in an article in *Diabetes Self-Management* (March/April 1993), explains that in the DCCT study this happened with almost half the people with long-standing diabetes. Intensive insulin therapy seems to accentuate the problem.

The physiological explanation for unawareness, according to Dinsmoor, is that people with diabetes lose the natural protections that keep blood sugar normal. These are the release of glucagon, which raises blood sugar, and epinephrine (also called adrenaline), which tells you with such symptoms as shaking and perspiring that it's down. Until something better comes long, the main solution is to monitor your blood sugar more frequently and *always* have glucose tablets available.

Why do I sometimes feel as if I'm having an insulin reaction when my blood sugar is normal?

It could be that physical or psychological factors unrelated to your diabetes are making you feel strange. But we have talked to several diabetics who maintain that they feel better with high blood sugar and that when it's normal they feel as if they're hypoglycemic.

Some of those who experience this phenomenon have been running around for quite a while with high blood sugar, either because they weren't testing their blood sugar and didn't realize how high it was or because they'd just been sloppy in their diabetes care. You know the song "I've Been Down So Long It Feels Like Up to Me"? Well, these diabetics have been up so long it feels like normal to them. Consequently, when they start bringing their blood sugar down to where it should be, they feel unnatural. It's almost like coming off a drug.

But if you stick to it and keep your blood sugar in the normal range, before long you'll feel right only when your blood sugar's right.

What do I do for an insulin reaction?

You eat or drink something sweet that will bring your blood sugar up fast. (This always confuses nondiabetics, who are convinced that diabetics can *never* have anything sugary and resist giving them what they need.) Most lists of what to eat for insulin reactions have been the same for years—and still are. They include a half glass of orange juice, sugar cubes, three or four Life Savers, a half cup of Coke or Pepsi, two tablespoons of raisins, etc. We've never understood how anyone could conceive of some of these items as handy to carry in your purse or pocket at all times. And we particularly don't fathom the magic of orange juice. It's actually low on the Carbohydrate Glycemic Index (46).

What you need in a low-blood-sugar emergency—and it should be treated as an emergency—is something quick and easy, good-tasting, and predictable. That's why we favor glucose tablets. Some of the more convenient ones are imported: Dextrosols (from England) and Dextro-Energens (from Germany). From the United States you have B-D Glucose Tablets, British American Medical's Dextrotabs, and Can-Am Cares's Dex 4's. All of these glucose tablets come in different flavors except B-D's. Dextrosols and Dex 4's will raise the blood sugar of a person weighing 120 to 150 pounds by approximately 15 milligrams per deciliter. Dextro-Energens raise blood sugar by 20 milligrams per deciliter and Dextrotabs by 8 milligrams per deciliter. The best way to find out exactly how much each of these tablets will raise *your* blood sugar is to test them on yourself. (Wait until your blood sugar is 100 or below; then eat one and retest in fifteen minutes.) If you know how many to eat for an insulin reaction, you won't make the classic mistake of overcompensating and sending yourself from 50 to 250. (This is called anxiety eating, and that term describes the phenomenon perfectly.)

If you get to the point where you are too far gone to chew but are conscious and able to swallow, the suggested treatment is one of the jels that can be absorbed in the mouth. These are Glutose (in a plastic container), Insta-Glucose (in a squeeze tube), and Monoject Insulin Reaction Gel (foil-wrapped pouch). A less expensive way to go is to pick up a few tubes of cake decorating icing in any supermarket.

Our final word: If you take insulin, live like a Boy Scout. Be prepared.

I've been told I should keep a supply of glucagon on hand. What is glucagon, and how is it used?

Glucagon is a hormone that's injected in the same way as insulin, only it has the opposite effect. It raises blood sugar. It's used to resuscitate diabetics who are unconscious because of low blood sugar.

Even if you never use it, glucagon is a nice security blanket. Just be sure whoever might be giving you an injection of glucagon knows where you keep it and how to administer it. And caution your family members or friends that if you're in insulin shock and unconscious, they should inject glucagon rather than trying to force liquid or food down your throat. An unconscious person cannot swallow and may choke to death.

Glucagon is available by prescription only. (This has never made sense to us, since insulin *isn't* a prescription medication and it's essential to have a supply of glucagon on hand if you take insulin.) It comes in the form of a Glucagon Emergency Kit made by Eli Lilly. A syringe is supplied and already filled with diluting solution which you mix with the powder. Many pharmacies do not regularly carry glucagon. When you find one that does or will order it for you, check the expiration date of glucagon; it should be about two years in advance. Prices can be very high, so comparison shop. (The kit is now around forty dollars.)

I'm afraid of having an insulin reaction when I'm asleep and never waking up. Can this happen?

This is so rare that we've heard of it happening only twice. One time it was a diabetic who went to bed drunk and wound up literally dead drunk. What happened was the alcohol suppressed the body's method of spontaneous recovery. Normally, the liver converts some of its stored starch to glucose, and that saves you. The moral of this story is to always go to bed sober.

The other instance was reported to us by the sister of a young man who died. She said he was so obsessively compulsive about never having a slightly elevated blood sugar that he always played it too close. One night he went to bed and didn't wake up. His sister found his blood-sugar record book and discovered that his before-bed blood sugar was 70. Obviously, he needed a snack before bed and either didn't have one or had too little. The moral of this story is not to be a fanatic about your blood-sugar control.

Many people wake up and feel restless when they have low blood sugar in the middle of the night. In this case, take your blood sugar and if it's low, eat glucose tablets and/or drink milk. (We hope you keep your meter at your bedside.) If you're experiencing more insulin reactions than usual, set your alarm for 2 a.m. and do a test. Your regimen may need changing. Have a snack before bed if your blood sugar is less than 120–150 or discuss with your doctor about altering your evening long-range insulin dose. With proper programming, a pump can easily solve this problem.

What is diabetic coma?

A diabetic coma occurs when your blood sugar is extremely high—perhaps over 1,000. You have diabetic ketoacidosis. Your sodium-bicarbonate and carbon-dioxide levels are low. You are dehydrated. Oddly enough, you don't have to be unconscious to be in diabetic coma. Only 15 percent of those in diabetic coma are.

To define it more bluntly, diabetic coma is what out-of-control diabetics die of. Death from diabetic coma has been totally preventable since the discovery of insulin in 1921.

To avoid getting yourself into this dangerous state:

- Do your best to always keep your diabetes under control.
- Never neglect testing your blood sugar. If it's high, test for ketones, too. If there are ketones, call your doctor.
- If you are insulin-dependent, never neglect taking your injection.
- Whenever you are ill, check with your doctor to see if you need to take more insulin.

Diabetic coma approaches slowly. The symptoms are thirst, frequent urination, fever, drowsiness, rapid breathing, vomiting or nausea, and finally unconsciousness. The treatment for ketoacidosis is regular insulin.

Can I get a driver's license if I take insulin?

Definitely yes. We don't know the regulations in all states, because they're all somewhat different, but we do know that the California Department of Motor Vehicles has liberal rules. Diabetics don't even have to reveal that they have diabetes unless they're subject to periods of unconsciousness.

Is it all right to drive a car alone on long trips?

Of course. You must, however, always carefully monitor your blood sugar. On *any* trip, short or long, never start out before checking your blood sugar and making sure it is normal or somewhat above normal. This should be a strict, no-exceptions-made personal law. We've heard of too many tragedies involving people with diabetes not to be fervent advocates of this policy. This is one of June's most inflexible rules, and she was lucky enough to learn it through other people's experience. Driving is dangerous enough without augmenting the risk with a fuzzy mind and an ill-coordinated body.

It goes without saying that you should have glucose tablets and snacks in the car with you. If you're on a long trip, stop at regular intervals (say, every hour) and test your blood sugar. Then you can snack enough to avoid low blood sugar. And if you take NPH or any other intermediate or long-acting insulin that programs you into certain eating hours, you should stop and eat when mealtime strikes. If you know there's a dearth of restaurants on the route or you're particular about what you eat, it's better to take along a picnic meal than to risk having to delay your meal or stoke up on snacks.

Is it okay to exercise alone if you take insulin?

It's always better to have a companion for safety's sake, as well as for company. You especially shouldn't do anything potentially hazardous like skiing or swimming alone.

Still, there isn't always somebody around, and a diabetic does always need exercise. There's no reason you can't take a walk or jog or ride your bicycle or play a round of golf by yourself. Just be sure you never leave the house without glucose tablets and enough snacks to see you through. *Enough* is the word here. Take along a lot more than you think you can possibly need. Then you'll never have to curtail your fun. Choose snacks that are good and, preferably, good for you, such as small packages of raisins or dried prunes, Fi-Bars, fruit leathers, trail mix, fruit-juice-sweetened cookies, peanut butter and crackers, and the like.

For People with Type II (Non-Insulin-Dependent) Diabetes

··

$\mathbf{I}$f you find Type II diabetes confusing and hard to understand, you're not alone. The general public doesn't understand it at all. What they think of when they hear the word "diabetes" is Type I, the kind in which you have to "stick yourself with a needle." They think this even though Type II's like you are in the vast majority—around 90 percent—of all people with diabetes. Many of them also erroneously think you got diabetes from eating too many sweets. The old "shame-on-you" factor kicks in.

Sad to say, there are also some health professionals who don't understand Type II diabetes very well either. Some even go so far as to consider Type II diabetes your fault. "If you weren't so overweight," they say judgmentally, "you wouldn't have diabetes." Here's another "shame-on-you" factor that's as wrong as it is cruel. (If you ever hear anything like this from a health professional, run, do not walk, out the door and never come back.)

And to make a personal confession for which we now hope to gain absolution, we, too, until recently totally misunderstood the true nature of Type II diabetes. We considered it "a kind of lifestyle disease" and even perpetuated the erroneous theory that "with

149

most Type II diabetics, diabetes is a symptom; the real disease is overweight." But in 1992 we became enlightened. We decided to write a book for Type II's whom we had finally come to consider the "neglected majority." Our collaborator and the person who set us straight once and for all was Virginia Valentine, R.N., C.D.E., and herself a not-thin Type II. Writing the book *Diabetes Type II and What to Do* was the educational process by which we learned what a complex and frustrating form of diabetes this is. Now we can pass our newfound knowledge on to you.

As we mentioned earlier, you were genetically programmed for this disease. It's extremely hereditary, much more so than Type I. If one twin gets Type I diabetes, it ain't necessarily so that the other will, too. If a twin gets Type II, though, the diagnosis of the other twin is almost invariably not far behind. In fact, we bet that if you climb around your family tree, you'll find you have a Type II diabetic up there somewhere—maybe on your own branch. This genetic programming for Type II makes your cells unreceptive to insulin. (Remember, insulin is like a key that unlocks the cells to let the glucose in to fuel the body.)

You were also genetically programmed to be overweight. You have thrifty genes that cause you to store calories more easily than those around you, even when you eat less than they do. This would make you a great survivor during a famine period or in a prison camp where they feed you a starvation diet, but it compounds your problem with your genetic disposition toward insulin resistance, since extra weight makes you even more resistant.

If you're a woman, you have another built-in weight-magnet. Women have a slower metabolism than men. If a man and a woman of the same general build eat the same number of calories and do the same amount of exercise, the woman is likely to put on weight while the man stays the same or even loses. This is nature's way of protecting pregnant women and their babies-to-be during times of low food supply. Nature can't seem to understand that you don't need this protection when you're neither pregnant nor starving. But at any rate, this slower metabolism is what helps make Type II diabetes more common in women than men.

Another general misconception is that all diabetics lack insulin. Again that's only true for Type I's. You probably have plenty of insulin, maybe even an excess amount. Your cells are just resistant to it or don't have enough receptors or both of the above. Your poor old pancreas keeps pumping out more insulin in a valiant effort to get those cells to open up and let the insulin and glucose do their thing. But it doesn't work. All that happens is that the insulin, which is a great fat-producing and storing hormone, makes you feel hungry all the time so you eat more and put on more weight and this makes your cells even more resistant and more and more sugar (glucose) is floating around your bloodstream. Since it can't get into the cells, your body stores a lot of this sugar as fat. This makes you even more insulin-resistant.

The last straw is that the liver, whose job it is to release glucose when it's needed by the body, gets the impression that it's time to do its job because, since no glucose is getting into the cells, it figures there must be no glucose in the bloodstream. (Obviously, the liver doesn't understand Type II diabetes very well either!) At any rate, the liver ("I'm just doing my job") pours forth glucose and your blood sugar goes ever higher. It goes so high that it is finally in the diabetic range. Ergo, you have Type II diabetes.

From all this, you can see it's not your fault that you have diabetes. As Virginia Valentine says loud and clear in *Diabetes Type II and What to Do,* "Diabetes is not a character flaw!"

What does it mean to be told you're a "borderline" diabetic?

It means the person who told you that has a very loose grasp on what diabetes is all about. There is no such thing as "borderline" diabetes. The term has been outmoded since 1979, when the National Diabetes Data Group came up with the Type I and Type II classifications of diabetes for insulin-dependent and non-insulin-dependent diabetes. Before that time Type I was called juvenile-onset, and Type II maturity-onset. Since age of onset of diabetes does not determine the type of diabetes (see page 154 about Type II children), these terms are considered misleading and inaccurate.

The new classification system also wiped out such fuzzy and often misunderstood terms as "chemical diabetes," subclinical diabetes," "asymptomatic diabetes," and "latent diabetes." All of these terms were replaced with "impaired glucose tolerance."

In a report published in the journal *Diabetes,* it was pointed out that impaired glucose tolerance is not diabetes and the use of the label "diabetes" for people with "marginal" blood levels "can invoke social, psychological, and economic sanctions that are unjustified in the light of the lack of severity of their glucose intolerance." (Translation: These people shouldn't be denied jobs that are forbidden to diabetics.)

The glucose-tolerance-test graph (Figure 1, page 153) shows the difference in glucose levels among a nondiabetic, a person with impaired glucose tolerance, and a diabetic.

As *Diabetes Forecast* points out, "while some people whose blood-glucose levels are somewhat elevated *do* develop diabetes, many people subsequently have normal tests and continue to test 'normal' indefinitely."

Our personal opinion is that if you have impaired glucose tolerance you should follow the diabetic lifestyle just to be on the safe side. But then we feel that *everybody* should follow the diabetic lifestyle.

I've heard that Type II diabetes isn't as serious as Type I diabetes. Is this true?

It's about as true as saying that if you forget about diabetes it will go away. We wish it were true, because then instead of 14 million diabetics in the United States there would be only 1 million. And we wish it were true for your sake, if you are a Type II, because that would mean you could relax and put your condition in the same category as a food allergy or a case of eczema.

No, it's not true. Type II diabetes is just as serious as Type I, and, like Type I, it will, if ignored or neglected, eventually cause health problems that are just as severe. The only difference is that the pattern of the development of these problems and their types may be somewhat different. Uncontrolled Type II diabetes leads most

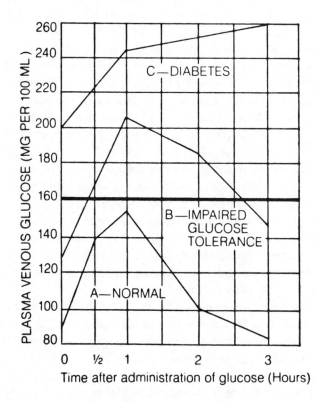

FIGURE 1. The three people represented on this graph each had 100 grams of glucose administered by mouth. One person (A-Normal) is nondiabetic. One person (B-Normal) has impaired glucose tolerance. And the other person (C-DM) is diabetic, either insulin-dependent or non-insulin-dependent. You can see that the nondiabetic's body has removed most of the glucose from circulation within two hours. In the diabetic, whose glucose levels were already too high, the glucose level shot even higher than at first, and three hours later the levels had not yet begun to drop. The person with impaired glucose tolerance has a curve similar to that of the nondiabetic, except that it is somewhat higher. Also, at the end of two hours this person's glucose level had dropped only slightly, whereas the nondiabetic's blood-glucose level had returned to normal. (*Courtesy of Gerald R. Cooper, M.D., Ph.D.,* Diabetes Forecast, *March–April 1980, p. 39. Copyright 1980 by the American Diabetes Association. Reprinted from* Diabetes Forecast *with permission.*)

often to heart disease, strokes, high blood pressure, and foot problems, while uncontrolled Type I diabetes is more likely to create eye, kidney, and nerve damage (in scientific terms, retinopathy, nephropathy, and neuropathy, respectively). Of course, Type II's can develop any of those complications also. In fact, Priscilla Hollander, M.D., writing in *Learning to Live Well with Diabetes,* says, "Neuropathy seems to appear earlier in people with Type II diabetes. In fact, it may be the first sign that a person has Type II diabetes."

A more positive piece of information is that these threats to your health do not develop fast. It takes eight or ten or even fifteen years for the body gradually to succumb to them. You do have to consider, however, that if you had high blood sugar several years before you were diagnosed diabetic, some damage could have been done before you were aware of your diabetes. This would explain why the development of neuropathy might be the first clue to your doctor that you have developed diabetes. As with many other diseases, the sooner you discover you have diabetes, the better off you are, because you can start normalizing your blood sugar and thereby prevent or reverse complications.

If you put two and two together you'll see that the leading complications of Type II diabetes are the same as those problems that tend to develop as you move into your more advanced years: heart disease, strokes, and high blood pressure. The most significant of these is high blood pressure. It's an astounding fact that between 45 and 50 percent of Type II's—regardless of their ethnic background or other risk factors—also have high blood pressure. The synergetic effect of Type II diabetes and aging can be worsened even more if your life-style has been and continues to be unhealthy (very little exercise, high-fat diet, smoking, etc.) and your family has a history of these diseases. All the more reason to play it safe and follow the life-style of the growing numbers of active, health-conscious seniors we now have in this country. And diabetes will show you the way.

Can children have Type II diabetes?

Here's the word from two authorities: Richard Guthrie, M.D., co-director of the Mid-America Diabetes Associates Program and director of the Diabetes Treatment Center at St. Joseph's Medical Center in Wichita, and Diana Guthrie, R.N., Ph.D., professor at the University of Kansas School of Medicine in Wichita.

> Overweight children with high blood-sugar levels are brought to our attention by referral from other physicians or parents who are concerned about the weight problem in the child. When we do a glucose-tolerance test on them, we also analyze for insulin values. These particular children, who usually have high glucose levels as well as high insulin values, return to normal laboratory values in most cases once weight loss has been achieved. We have not followed them to find out about complications, but we have seen some children in this descriptive category become Type II diabetics. The main treatment, of course, is increasing the activity level with the ultimate goal of decreasing the weight. Usually, the children are not on restricted caloric intake, but we work very strongly with maintaining the caloric intake and increasing the activity level.

Since I don't take insulin, do I have to do all that blood-sugar testing?

Absolutely. All diabetics who want to keep normal blood-sugar levels, and that should be your goal, have to test their blood sugar to assure themselves that they are staying on track. No way out. Well, there is an illusory way out. You may have been put on old-fashioned urine-sugar testing instead of blood-sugar testing and led to believe that if there is no sugar in your urine, your blood sugar is okay. Supposedly, no sugar in the urine means you are staying under 180—the normal renal threshold, as it is called. It is the normal level at which sugar moves into the urine in a desperate attempt to keep you out of what Dr. Peter Forsham calls "glucotoxicity" (sugars high enough to poison your system).

But this is the rub: since most people are older when diagnosed and the renal threshold goes up with age, finding no sugar in your urine may simply mean that your renal threshold has edged up. But your blood sugar might still be dangerously high. This is common with older Type II's who may have been introduced to urine testing years ago when it was the only test you could take.

For example, we talked to the daughter of a diabetic woman who, according to her daughter, "*loves* to eat, especially at big family gatherings." The mother would take her urine test, it would show that she wasn't spilling sugar, and so, presuming her blood sugar to be normal, she'd sit down happily and, as her daughter put it, "have a feast."

The woman wound up in the hospital with dangerous ketoacidosis. She'd been running extremely high blood sugar, but it had never shown up in her urine because of her high renal threshold.

This woman is now testing her blood sugar regularly at home. She doesn't have many feasts these days, but she's going to be around for a lot more normal meals than she would have been had she continued to dwell in a diabetes fool's paradise with her urine tests.

Another insidious aspect about being casual with your self-care and testing is that if you run around too long with elevated blood sugar, those diabetes complications we're always talking about can start slowly and quietly developing. You may never even know what is going on until the damage is done. We're not fear-mongers, and we don't like to threaten you with the problems diabetics are heir to, but in our experience many non-insulin-dependent diabetics don't get the point about the seriousness of diabetes the way insulin takers do.

Remember that even if you don't take insulin, you have to be as careful as if you did. Actually, Type II's are the most likely candidates for arrival at the hospital with diabetes-related complications or, as Professor Diana Guthrie warns, "to have to have part of a leg removed," because they're the ones most likely to ignore their diabetes until it screams for attention.

My doctor has prescribed pills to help me control my blood-sugar levels. What are these, and are they safe?

They are oral drugs that help lower blood sugar in some Type II diabetics. They are not oral insulin, as some people think. (Insulin cannot effectively be taken orally, as it is a protein and is digested.) These drugs have a twofold effect. They encourage your pancreas to make more insulin and they make your cells more receptive to insulin.

These oral hypoglycemics, as the doctors call them, all belong to one class of drugs, the sulfonylureas. The first generation of sulfonylureas (known generically as tolbutamide, chlorpropamide acetohexamide, and tolazamide) carry an FDA warning about their causing an increased risk of heart attack (just what you don't need). The second generation of oral hypoglycemics (generically called glyburide and glipizide), which came into use in the United States in 1984, are much more potent and are considered safer in that they cause fewer side effects because the dosage is smaller and they do not interact with other drugs. Table 4 shows the entire choice of sulfonylurea drugs now available.

TABLE 4.
Oral Hypoglycemics

Generic Name	Trade Name	Available Dosage Strengths, Tablets (mg)	Maximum Dosage (gm/day)	Duration Action (hours)
FIRST GENERATION				
Tolbutamide	Orinase	250–500	2.0–3.0	6–12
Chlorpropamide	Diabinese	100–250	0.5	up to 600
Acetohexamide	Dymelor	250–500	1.5	12–24
Tolazamide	Tolinase	100–250–500	1.5	10–16
SECOND GENERATION				
Glyburide	Micronase®	1.25–2.5 to 5	20 mg	18–30
Glyburide	Diabeta®	1.25–2.5 to 5	20 mg	18–30
Glipizide	Glucotrol®	5 to 10	40 mg	14–20

There is a new oral agent, Obinese (a combination of Diabinese and Metformin), but as of this writing it is not available in the U.S. although it can be obtained in both Mexico and Canada. Some Type II's who failed to keep their blood sugars in control on the other pills have been able to lower their blood sugars another 50 or 60 points on Obinese and thereby get along without insulin at least for a while longer.

Oral-drug therapy is a next-to-the-last-resort treatment for Type II diabetes. The first line of defense is diet and exercise. Then if blood sugars do not retreat, the person is a candidate for some kind of pill. If pills alone don't cause improvement, you can take advantage of a new technique being tried: combining pills with one shot of insulin a day, usually a small amount of intermediate-acting NPH at bedtime. The disadvantage here is that the insulin may increase obesity.

If you are using oral drugs, you do need to monitor your blood sugar on a regular basis. Since the advent of the newer, stronger oral drugs, you must watch particularly for low blood sugar. The second-generation drugs are likely to cause more hypoglycemia, because they are more effective. If you use one of them, eat your meals regularly and check your blood sugar when you exercise or when you have symptoms of hypoglycemia: sweating, shaking, dizziness, slurred speech, blurred vision, hunger, irritability, nausea, or confusion. Glipizide is probably the best choice for an older person since it is less likely to cause hypoglycemia.

You also need to check your blood sugar, because many people have what is known as "secondary failure" on their oral drug. Sixty percent of the people who initially got good results with first-generation pills, which have been used in the United States for thirty-two years, failed on them after six years. The hope is that this experience won't be repeated with the second-generation drugs.

Obviously, if you fail on the pills the next step is insulin.

Insulin?! I thought I had non-insulin-dependent diabetes. Why are we talking about insulin?

A lot of people believe that Type II's never have to take insulin unless they take it temporarily when they're ill or have surgery or some other stress to the body. Unfortunately, a lot of people are wrong. The truth, according to our Type II guru, Virginia Valentine, is that "as many as 25 to 50 percent of Type II's will eventually be using insulin to manage their diabetes."

The first step in Type II management is keeping your blood sugar in control, using diet and exercise. If that works, fine. You have the best of all possible Type II worlds. If it *doesn't* work, or if it works for a while and then works no more, the next step is to use the pills we were just discussing. These usually keep your blood sugar in the proper range for an average of five to seven years, although Virginia Valentine reports having one patient who's been successfully on the pills for twenty-five years.

Then, if the time comes that your physician decides that your blood sugars aren't what they should be—say, your fasting (before-breakfast) blood sugars are over 150 and your after-meal blood sugars are over 200, then it's time to call in the old master blood-sugar controller, insulin.

You may protest at this point, "I thought you said that I probably had lots of insulin floating around in my bloodstream—maybe even too much." You probably did have plenty of insulin. That's *did.* Past tense. Over the years your poor pancreas has been working overtime. Now it's weary. It can no longer produce enough insulin to keep your blood sugar in the acceptable range, so you have to help it out by bringing some more insulin on board.

Maybe your doctor will give you a combination of pills and a small amount of NPH—intermediate-acting—insulin at bedtime to see if that does the job. Other doctors believe that once the pills stop working you shouldn't use them anymore at all and will put you directly onto insulin alone.

Many Type II's who go onto insulin are put on only one shot of NPH a day. That's usually not a good idea because it probably won't keep you in control for the entire twenty-four hours. One of the better insulin-therapy programs currently being used is to take two shots a day of a combination of premixed 70 percent NPH and 30 percent regular (fast-acting) insulin. This combination usually covers you all day and night and takes care of your after-meal blood-sugar rises as well.

We know you don't like reading about taking insulin. You don't even like to think about it. But really, taking insulin is not as bad as it sounds. Most people who've built it up into a horrifying monster are surprised that it's not such a big deal once they get into doing it. Actually, it even has a couple of advantages beyond the obvious ones of keeping your blood sugar normal and preventing complications. (1) It costs a lot less than the pills and (2) If you take insulin, Medicare and those insurance plans that cover only what Medicare does will pay for your blood-sugar meter and strips, whereas if you don't take insulin, they won't.

Since overweight is such a problem for Type II's, how can I lose weight quickly, easily, and permanently?

That's a big question as well as an important one. It's so big and important, in fact, that we've added a whole section on weight loss to the end of the book. See the chapter "How to Win at Losing."

Everyone talks about people with Type II diabetes having to lose weight. I was diagnosed in my 40s and told I have Type II and yet I've never been overweight in my life. In fact, I've usually been underweight. What am I supposed to do?

We know just how you feel. Your story is June's story. She was diagnosed at age forty-five and told she had Type II diabetes and she was thin at the time. After trying to make it on the pills for a year she was actually gaunt because she'd been out-of-control for so long. When she went onto insulin—where she should have been in the first place—she regained her normal weight and health.

She and you are what is sometimes called Type I ½, or what Virginia Valentine calls Type II-D, meaning deficient. That's because you're deficient in insulin. (She calls the other Type II's type II-R's because they're insulin resistant.)

You have one foot in each diabetes world. You can be called Type II because you were diagnosed in mid-to-late life, when most of them were. But then you could also be called Type I because your pancreas doesn't produce enough insulin, so you'll have to take some insulin (better sooner rather than later like June). You won't, however, have to take as much as most true Type I's because you do produce some insulin of your own. Unlike Type II-R's, your cells aren't resistant to insulin and you don't have a lot of insulin floating around in your bloodstream knocking on the cell doors trying to get in.

What June does is treat herself pretty much as if she were a Type I, but she cherishes the knowledge that with her (and your) kind of middle-of-the-road diabetes, you do better at avoiding the complications of diabetes. (June has no complications after twenty-seven years of diabetes.) That's because producing some of your own insulin seems to be a protective feature against the Type I complications, and not having excessive insulin in your bloodstream the way Type II-R's do reduces the cardiovascular risks of their kind of diabetes. That small amount of insulin that you produce also makes it a little easier for you to control your blood sugar than the classic Type I that produces none.

This doesn't mean that you can just relax and let your special kind of diabetes take care of itself. You still have to care for yourself and your disease just as meticulously as the other two more clear-cut types.

Watch out for one thing, though, especially when you're first diagnosed. Don't let anyone hand you a diet sheet and tell you to lose some weight and shove you out the door. We've known it to happen more than once.

And here's another terrific advantage for you. You get to read both the Type I and Type II sections of this book and pick and choose which parts apply to your kind of diabetes. How's that for luck?!

For Family and Friends

. . . .

They say that one person in four is touched by diabetes. That is to say, you have it, you eventually will have it, or you are a family member or close friend of someone who has it. Since you're reading this section, you probably fall into one of the two latter categories. And you have your problems, too.

June, in her more mellow moments, allows that she thinks diabetes is sometimes harder on family members and friends of diabetics than on the diabetics themselves. She may be right, especially when it comes to the parents of diabetic children. For many of them their guilt feelings, anguish, and constant worry are exquisite torture. Parents often lie awake fretting through the night while in the next room their diabetic child sleeps—appropriately enough—like a baby.

Some adult diabetics manage to lay all the responsibility for their care on a spouse. In these cases it's usually—but certainly not always—the wife of a diabetic who learns the diabetic diet, prepares it, and tries to see to it that her husband sticks to it while he remains aloof and unconcerned. On the other hand, we had a husband drop by a SugarFree Center who did the blood-sugar testing for his diabetic wife. He took the blood sample, read it, recorded the results—in short, handled everything—because she refused to have anything to do with it.

Friends of those with diabetes sometimes encounter the opposite situation. The diabetic person doesn't want to impose his or her problem on someone else and so will hardly talk about it, let alone clue in the friend on how to help on a day-to-day basis or even in time of emergency.

It's never easy. In a sense family members and friends are like insulin-taking diabetics who walk a tightrope between high and low blood sugar. Only the tightrope you walk is between not doing enough and doing too much, between being oblivious to a diabetic's problems and being concerned to the point of driving the diabetic—and yourself—crazy.

In this section we'll try to help you with your delicate and nerve-racking balancing act and show you that although you're touched by diabetes, you don't have to be pushed around, pummeled, and knocked out by it.

By the way, it's a good idea for you to read *all* the questions in this section, even the ones that on the surface don't appear to apply to you. You may find just the help you need buried in a seemingly unrelated situation.

Will diabetes make changes in our family life?

Only about as many changes as moving a hippopotamus into the living room. Each looms large on the scene, can't be ignored, has to be worked around, demands a great deal of time and trouble and care; and you never stop wishing that someone would take the damned thing away.

But strangely enough, you can get used to anything, be it hippopotamus or diabetes. Eventually when people express shock and concern—"Oh, you have a hippopotamus in your living room!" (or "Oh, your child, husband, or wife has diabetes!") "How terrible!"—you're surprised they even mention it as an oddity or a problem. It's just what *is,* a part of your life—and you're living with it.

How do I help the diabetic person in my life?

Learn. Learn all you can about diabetes. Become a walking encyclopedia of diabetes lore so you can be an intelligent and informed as well as a caring partner. Notice we say *partner*. Don't do it all. Don't try to take over. Don't make the diabetic—child or adult—totally dependent on you. That's not an act of kindness. People with diabetes have to be responsible for themselves. After all, you can't be around every minute—and even if you can you shouldn't be.

It's especially important for you to attend diabetes education classes and diabetes-association meetings with the diabetic person. Not only does this give emotional support, but two sets of eyes and ears absorbing the information make the program twice as effective.

If you have a diabetic child, we especially recommend that you join the Juvenile Diabetes Foundation International (see Reference Section: Directory of Organizations). Their primary goal is the worthy one of raising funds to finance research toward a cure for diabetes. But membership in this organization has the additional value of putting you in touch with other parents of diabetic children with whom you can share problems and—more important—solutions.

Another way to learn about diabetes is somewhat unusual, but if you're up to doing it, it will increase your understanding of diabetes tremendously and also help you develop empathy for the diabetic. Empathy is better than sympathy. Sympathy is feeling sorry for people; empathy is feeling how they feel, almost getting inside their skin.

Here's the way: you live exactly as a diabetic lives for a period of time. This idea was developed at the Diabetic Unit of the Queen Elizabeth II Medical Center in Western Australia, where they believed that the staff who treated diabetics needed to know what their patients' lives were really like. Volunteers for the experiment were required to take injections, using a saline solution instead of insulin, test their blood, eat the diabetic diet, including snacks at the proper time, etc. These educators had to "be diabetic" for only a week, but some of them couldn't last even that long. The only one who was really successful at it just gave up her social life entirely and stayed at home catering to her diabetes. That, of course, isn't the way to do it. You're supposed to lead a normal life. After all, that's the goal for diabetics, and that's what everyone else is always telling them they can do.

As Dr. Martyn Sulway, the physician in charge of the program, put it, "They found out having diabetes isn't a piece of cake." (Australian pronunciation: "pace of kaike.")

Barbara, even though she thought she knew all she needed to about the diabetic life, decided to try the experiment, because she'd been haranguing diabetics for years about what they ought to do yet had no firsthand experience. She did it, not for a week but for a month. It was a revelation.

Although she'd always bragged about eating the diabetes diet, she discovered that she hadn't been nearly as meticulous about it as a diabetic needs to be. For example, she hadn't always turned down *every* dessert. Also, she hadn't had to be continually worrying about keeping the inexorable snack on hand for an emergency, *and*—this irritated her the most—she hadn't had to eat when she wasn't hungry.

She took twice-daily blood sugars (and to her surprise discovered that she may have a twinge of reactive hypoglycemia). She took three injections a day. In order to have a little health hype out of it, she shot vitamin B_{12} instead of saline solution. Strangely enough, the injections weren't as bad as expected. At first they were an interesting novelty, but before long they became just a bore. Occasionally and for no apparent reason the shots hurt, but most of the time they were relatively painless.

She even managed to get the flu (not deliberately) and decided that if she really had been diabetic she would have wound up in the hospital because her diabetes-care program fell totally to pieces. This really brought home how important it is for a diabetic to avoid getting the minor diseases that go around every year.

Barbara also developed a greater tolerance for the foibles and peccadillos of diabetics. She has always been aghast at reports that some teenagers (and even one diabetic celebrity) shoot through their clothes when out in restaurants. But one night during the first week of the experiment she was dining out with friends and suddenly realized halfway through the meal that she'd forgotten to take her "insulin." So *zap!*—right through the old corduroy pants and into the leg.

One of the worst features of "having diabetes," Barbara found, was having to keep your mind cluttered with it every minute.

As June says, it's as if you're always playing an intricate chess game on top of whatever else you're doing.

The *truly* worst feature of diabetes—the worry about hypoglycemia and long-term complications—can't be duplicated in a nondiabetic person. Still, you can learn an amazing amount.

Why should I follow the diabetic diet and exercise plan?

It will help keep your diabetic loved one doing it. But that's not the main reason. The main reason is that it will maintain your own good health. There's nothing peculiar about the diabetic life-style. It's what we all should be doing. If you read the recommendations for good health from the Department of Agriculture and Department of Health and Human Services, or the American Heart Association, you'll see they're nothing more than the well-balanced meals with fresh fruits and vegetables, whole grains, no concentrated sweets, and reduced fats recommended for diabetics. The diabetes exercise program, too—regular amounts of aerobic exercise—is exactly what everyone should be doing, according to all fitness experts.

Actually, having a diabetic person in your life or home is a tremendous boon. It wakes the entire family up to the best way of living and gives them an incentive for doing it.

It's particularly valuable when there are nondiabetic children in the family. If a sister or brother or parent has diabetes and the house is therefore bereft of junk food, they're going to develop healthy eating habits that will stay with them all through life.

Then, too, if any of the nondiabetics have the genetic gun loaded with a diabetic tendency, leading the diabetic lifestyle may well keep the trigger from ever being pulled.

And here's what may be the most effective inducement: If you have a diabetic spouse and he or she follows the diet and exercise program and you don't, you won't be able to measure up to your youthfully lean and vital counterpart. This can be bad for the dynamics of the marriage, to say nothing of your ego.

We feel compelled to warn you, however, of a built-in hazard when you're a nondiabetic in the company of a diabetic. That hazard is the old slip twixt the cup (and the fork and the spoon) and the lip. In other words, although you know better, you are constantly tempted to eat for two, and, alas, you often succumb to that temptation.

Here's how it works. The well-behaved diabetic is eye-measuring his or her food at a meal and eating right on the diet. You're doing pretty much the same, or maybe you're eating a *little* more, because after all you don't have to be all that careful with your measurements.

Then it turns out there are leftovers. They'll never be so tasty again. In fact, it would be foolish to try to keep them. And you don't want to waste all that good food. Think of the starving people around the world. So . . . down the hatch.

A few hours pass, and if the diabetic takes insulin it's time for a snack because he or she has to have small amounts of food at regular intervals to feed the insulin. As long as the diabetic is munching you figure you might as well be companionable and munch along. Your snack, which, again, doesn't have to be so carefully measured, goes down the hatch.

Dining out is even more tempting and hazardous. Perhaps there's a bottle of wine and the diabetic permits him- or herself one three-ounce glass. Somebody has to drink the rest. It cost a lot of money. You can't send it back, and they don't have doggie bags for liquids. Down the hatch.

Maybe there's a really fantastic dessert selection and the dessert comes with the meal. The diabetic prudently says no. Two desserts go down the hatch.

When you and the diabetic are at a friend's home for dinner, your eating for two becomes almost a social necessity. The hostess has worked so very hard on hors d'oeuvres and exotic concoctions—especially exotic dessert concoctions—that she's going to be wounded right down to the bottom of her saucepan if *someone* doesn't lap up with gusto everything in sight and ask for more. The diabetic can't. It's up to you. Down the hatch.

If this keeps up, before too long that hatch of yours is going to be attached to a tub, a tub that is in imminent danger of sinking. This is especially true if the diabetic person in your life is a relative, such as a sister or brother, with whom you share the same heredity. In this case, with your eating for two you could chomp your way into Diabetesland.

You have been warned. If you don't want that long and healthy life insurance policy your diabetic loved one has provided for you canceled, you have to pay the premium. That premium is to exert the same self-control as he or she and eat for only one. Then close down the hatch.

Should I marry someone with diabetes?

That, like the decision to marry at all, has ultimately to be your own decision, as you undoubtedly well know. The probable reason for asking this is that you're concerned about the problems your potential mate's diabetes might cause in the future.

It's wise to think about these possible problems now rather than later. As diabetes teaching nurse Diane Victor said to a young man who was complaining about some aspect of his wife's diabetes and shirking his responsibility for helping to deal with it, "Look, you knew she was diabetic when you married her. You signed on for the duration. Shape up."

Diabetes is never problem free, as we've made clear in this book and as you have probably already personally observed if you have a close relationship with a diabetic. Diabetes care takes time, time you would prefer to spend on more entertaining activities. Diabetes care takes money, money you would prefer to spend on other things. For a woman, diabetes can make having children more difficult, hazardous, and—again—expensive. And diabetes, if not cared for properly and controlled, can eventually cause debilitating complications and an earlier death.

But all of this doesn't mean you should give back (or take back) the engagement ring. Marriage is full of risks. You could marry a flawless specimen bearing a doctor's certificate of perfect health and the day after your wedding he or she or even you could get in an accident that paralyzed everything south of the earlobes. We have a friend whose apparently healthy wife developed multiple sclerosis in the first year they were married.

There are no guarantees in life. When you get married, the old "for better or for worse; in sickness and in health" still holds true. Realistically considered, diabetes, if well controlled, is one of the lesser worses and healthier sicknesses, and knowing about it in advance gives you a chance to learn and prepare and adjust.

Of course, it is possible for diabetes to destroy a marriage. Some marriages are so tenuous that they can't survive any adversity. In such cases, if it hadn't been diabetes that caused the breakup, something else would have.

Diabetes can also strengthen marriages. When one partner develops a potentially life-threatening condition, this makes the other realize how important the previously taken-for-granted person really is. Working together to control diabetes can, in fact, bring a new closeness. We heard of a long-married couple whose children had grown and who had gradually become so consumed by their individual interests that they hardly had anything left in common. Each was running on a separate track. When the wife was diagnosed diabetic, the tracks merged as they headed toward the same goal.

In the final analysis we believe that love conquers all. By this we don't mean the short-lived romantic love that turns your mind to irrational (but delicious) mush. No, we're referring to the enduring, day-to-day growing love that comes from living through and living with problems together and helping each other play out whatever hands you may be dealt, trying to turn the game into a winning one.

Does a diabetic child disrupt a family?

A diabetic child can disrupt it or can merely change it, in some ways for the better. Disruptions occur when the parents are filled with guilt, anger, or both. We heard of a husband who blamed his wife for the child's diabetes and threatened to divorce her "if anything happens to that kid." Obviously, he hadn't heard of the theory of the cause of Type I diabetes being a virus, just as the cause of the measles or mumps is a virus.

Parents fraught with guilt can coddle and overindulge a diabetic child. This not only creates resentment and feelings of being unloved in any other children in the family but can be ruinous for the diabetic child as well. Diabetes can become for the child an excuse for dependence and manipulation of other family members instead of a stepping-stone to strength.

On the other hand, psychologist Barbara Goldberg, writing in *Diabetes Forecast,* emphasized that every family of a diabetic child that she talked to "mentioned that, in spite of, or perhaps because of, the illness, there was a special protectiveness, helpfulness, and a greater sense of family closeness."

This also holds true if one parent becomes diabetic. In American families these days we tend to be more than somewhat child centered. If a parent becomes diabetic and needs attention and care from the rest of the family, this develops in the children an increased responsibility and sensitivity to the needs of others.

In one family, the father, who had flexible business hours, spent much of his spare time chauffeuring the kids to their many and varied sporting activities and cheering them on from the sidelines. When he developed diabetes and had a need for exercise himself, the kids made it their business to see that dad got his jog every day and took turns accompanying him on it. New responsibilities. New closeness.

What can I do for my diabetic child?

There are many things you can do. You can help the child accept the disease and teach him or her how to take care of it. You can encourage diabetic children to achieve whatever they want to achieve in life despite diabetes. But there's one extremely important thing parents sometimes fail to do because they don't know it needs to be done— help diabetic children get rid of some of the terrible fears they carry around inside and suffer over and don't talk about.

Dr. Robert Rood, a San Fernando Valley diabetologist who works with children and adolescents, told a story about a child at a summer camp where he was serving as physician. This girl was a model camper, full of fun and very popular.

Dr. Rood, in checking out her blood tests, discovered that her one shot of insulin a day wasn't doing the job. (These were the bad old days when one shot a day was typical.) He decided to divide her insulin into two doses—morning and evening. This worked fine.

Her blood sugar returned to normal. But *she* became very *ab*normal—sullen, negative, picking fights. When he took her aside to talk, she broke down and started crying. "I don't want to die," she said between sobs.

"Die?" said Dr. Rood. "Why are you talking about dying?"

"I know my diabetes was bad before when I had to take one shot. *Now* it must be getting lots worse because I have to take two. I'm going to die. I know it."

Dr. Rood reassured her, of course, and she became her old self again, but he had learned something important. You never know what's going on in a child's head. You have to take the time to talk and explain. Be especially careful if there are any major changes in diabetes routines, lest the child interpret them as Dr. Rood's camper did.

Diabetic children also sometimes believe their diabetes is a punishment for "being bad." This gives them guilt feelings as well as fear if they're ever "bad" again something even worse will happen.

And don't overlook the hidden fears and guilts of the nondiabetic children in the family. Younger children can get the idea that when they reach the age when the older child got it, they'll get diabetes, too. Each day to them becomes like the tick of a time bomb.

Guilt feelings arise when nondiabetic children have harbored some quite normal sibling-rivalry evil thoughts, like "I wish Eddie would die," and lo, Eddie gets diabetes. They hold themselves responsible.

Parents must be aware of these dangers when the element of diabetes enters the family. Diabetes means there must be closer communication, more understanding, and more openness in the family. And that's all to the good.

If my diabetic child goes to a birthday party or trick-or-treating on Halloween, is it all right to break the diet just this once?

Think how many "just this once's" that would make in a year. Before long, just this once becomes an everyday occurrence and bad habits are established. Your child's health and maybe even life expectancy are diminished.

It's hard to see your child deprived when other kids are loading up on goodies—maybe it's even harder on you than on the child—but diabetes is going to be there all his or her life. Now is when lifetime behavior patterns are established. You're *not* being kind when you let your child break his or her diet just this once.

One thing you can do on occasions when your child is being deprived is figure out some way he or she can get extra attention. Attention is an even more satisfying commodity to the young (or the middle-aged and old, for that matter) than ice cream, cake, and candy. Let your child pass out the forbidden food to others in much the same way that some alcoholics like to act as bartender at parties.

You can also give parties at your own home. That allows you to present approved food in such entertaining ways that neither your child nor the guests will realize, or care, that they aren't getting the junk food their hearts desire.

As for Halloween, your first decision is whether to allow your child out at all. If you do, and he or she comes home with a bag of loot, ADA board member Netti Richter, writing in *Diabetes Forecast,* offers some good suggestions:

> Why not help sort out the acceptable healthy foods and save a few sugary ones for handling reactions? What about the rest of the candy? In our house the garbage disposal is a great eater of "nondesirable foods."
>
> Knowing that resisting candy will be rewarded by an exchange gift at evening's end might make trick-or-treating less frustrating for a child. For example, exchanging the candy for a Halloween storybook at bedtime can be fun.

Use your own imagination to help your child stay on the diet instead of using your pity to allow him or her to break it "just this once."

Now, after having given the official party line, which happens to be our own opinion as well, here's a more lenient variation reported by a physician whom we respect, Dr. Lawrence Power, author of the syndicated column "Food and Fitness" and consulting physician for National Health Systems (publishers of health reference charts).

A colleague of his who sees many diabetic children and young people says that a number of young diabetics, especially teenagers, who don't want to be different and who long for the fun foods their peers get to wolf down, totally rebel. They refuse to follow their diets and as a result stay constantly out of control.

This doctor makes a deal with the kids. If they promise to stick to their diet at all other times, they get six Hog Wild Days a year, six celebration days such as Christmas or their birthdays or graduation day, when, as far as food is concerned, anything goes.

"Do you know how high they usually kick up their heels on those days?" the doctor asks. "A Coke and a hamburger or a hot fudge sundae. Big deal."

Dr. Power himself adopted the Hog Wild Day method with his adult heart-attack patients. "Everyone needs a binge now and then," he says, "whether it's mint bonbons, Big Macs, or a cholesterol quiche. Something in most of us calls for a break from the routine. . . . There's room for the occasional departure for a holiday. It is the daily habits that get us into health mischief, not the occasional celebration."

Only you know your child well enough to decide whether the Hog Wild system would be a safety valve that would let off enough steam to allow him or her to simmer down to a good daily dietary routine or if it would only break down the already flimsy barriers against hazardous eating habits.

If you *do* opt for Hog Wildness, you should have a clear understanding with your child that the six days are to be spread out over the year and not clustered into an orgy week that could prove disastrous.

Should I send my child to diabetes summer camp?

Unless your child is the kind who would be miserably homesick and suffer psychological damage at *any* summer camp, we think it's a good idea—especially for younger and newly diagnosed children. We've had reports from young people who consider their camp experience a breakthrough in understanding their diabetes and in learning new practical techniques of management. Even more important to them was the realization that they're not oddballs and that the world is full of other diabetic children who are successfully coping with the condition.

It's a genuine comfort for a diabetic person to be in a situation in which virtually everyone has diabetes and the person *without* diabetes is the peculiar one. Barbara experienced this one day back when we ran the SugarFree Centers. June and Ron, both diabetic, were on the scene, as was our cleaning woman, also diabetic. (We practiced reverse discrimination and hired diabetic employees whenever we could.) Everyone who came in had diabetes. All the mail was from people with diabetes. Barbara began to get the creepy feeling that she was the only nondiabetic person on earth and that there was something wrong with her for *not* having it.

Summer camp is also a good way for a child who has perhaps been overprotected at home because of diabetes to develop self-reliance.

One major benefit of diabetes summer camp is for the parents. For a short while you get out from under the stress and strain of worrying about your diabetic child. You know he or she is in the best of hands and you can get away for a little R and R yourself. You need it and you deserve it. Stress works its damage on you as well as on the diabetic child.

Summer camp can also give you a chance to improve your relationship with any nondiabetic children in the family. They may be developing feelings of being less loved because they don't get the constant concern that the diabetic child gets. A week or two of exclusive attention can be a booster shot of security and self-esteem for them.

We have heard a few complaints about diabetes summer camps, including one from a mother whose already too-thin child came home five pounds lighter and showing ketones, and from a young woman who was disturbed and disgusted by the wild goings-on with alcohol and marijuana in one camp for teenagers. But these are isolated instances. The overwhelming majority of the reports have been favorable.

What can we do if we can't afford all the costs involved with our child's diabetes?

There is help available in the form of Supplemental Security Income (SSI). This is a federal program that makes monthly cash payments to disabled people who don't own much in the way of property or other assets and who don't have much income. Diabetes counts as a disability. A child's SSI payment can be as much as $477 a month, although some may get less because of their parents' income.

For further information, and for instructions on how to file, call the SSI office at 1-800-772-1213.

I just can't get my husband to take care of his diabetes no matter how hard I try. Is there anything I can do?

Unfortunately, you're not alone. Many people are desperate about trying to get those they love to take care of their diabetes and themselves. We frequently receive letters like the following, written by a young man:

> I have been involved with a wonderful lady name Sheila. About a year and a half ago we learned that she is a Type I diabetic. We are always considering marriage, but I must admit I'm frightened about our future together. Her problem is not the fact that she is diabetic. She has been fighting a losing battle with a severe sugar addiction. It has nearly destroyed our relationship many times, and she becomes so depressed that it is really unbearable. She desperately wants to beat this addiction to sweets, but nothing has seemed to work for more than a day or two at a time. There is some progress, but I fear that time is quickly running out. Sheila has already noticed a decrease in her vision as well as constant poor circulation. Her diabetologist dropped her as a patient because she was not doing what he told her. It's evident that these sugar binges of hers could prove fatal.

> I love Sheila with all my heart and soul and want so much to beat this damned disease and have as much of a future as God would permit us. Such a wonderful person as Sheila deserves as full a life as possible. I hope she can take control of this disease before it takes control of her.

We also get success stories. We received this note attached to a law school graduation announcement: "We got our meter in December. Since then my husband's diabetes has been controlled. It certainly took a load of worry off my mind during my last year in law school. In that light I wanted to share my graduation with you."

One young woman confessed to us that her husband told her that she used to be disagreeable about half the time, but since she started controlling her blood sugar, she's become "a wonderful human being and a joy to be around."

You might have your husband read the above so he could see what a shattering—or positive—effect a diabetic's control can have on loved ones. You could express your feelings. Even if he isn't willing to control the diabetes for himself, he might start doing it to free you and the rest of the family from worry and allow you all to live your lives to the fullest.

But if people with diabetes should decide to control their blood sugar for the benefit of others, they should also investigate why they don't want to control it for themselves. Don't they consider themselves worth the effort? Don't they love themselves enough? If the answer is no, they may have a real problem, a problem more serious than diabetes and one for which they should seek professional counseling.

But if your husband still won't take care of himself, remember that it is as Dr. Richard R. Rubin says: "Nobody can make anyone else do something they don't want to do." He advises you to "recognize, grieve, and finally accept the reality of your own limits." But still, "you should never stop trying new ways of helping the person locate his or her own motivation for change."

What is this "honeymoon period" I hear about?

This can occur in Type I diabetes—particularly in children—shortly after insulin treatment begins. The diabetes seems to be in remission. Less insulin, or sometimes none at all, is needed for diabetes control. This often causes parents who are already desperately clutching at straws to think their child has been miraculously cured or that the diagnosis was wrong. False hope. Diabetes is still there. A remission is not a cure and should never be regarded as such. Enjoy it while it lasts, but realize that it will end, and don't let yourself be devastated when it does.

My wife wants to think and talk about diabetes all the time. What can I do?

It's hard to find a person with diabetes who's middle-of-the-road. Either they try to ignore the disease totally or become almost obsessed by it. Those who fall into the obsessive category are at least better than the ignorers. They'll probably live longer and eventually outgrow their obsession.

As a matter of fact, many people are obsessed only for a while, right after they're diagnosed. It's not surprising that they should be preoccupied when they first confront a disease that demands the constant attention and thought that diabetes does. Much of the diabetic's talk about diabetes at this time is just musing out loud as he or she tries to figure out what to do.

One way that might tone the diabetic decibels down a little is to become more informed about diabetes yourself. By showing that you know something about the subject, your wife may begin to feel less desperate about the subject and relax and let you do some of the thinking. If the two of you have workable give-and-take exchanges on new solutions to diabetic problems, perhaps she will be able to cut the personal, lonely fretting time in half and start to think and talk about something else.

Your advantage in knowing about diabetes is that when it's the subject under discussion, you'll understand what's being said. Then the talking will seem a lot less like a foreign language you don't speak, and consequently, it will become a lot less boring to you.

If this plan doesn't work or just seems to feed the obsession, you may eventually have to express a little tough love. Say in no uncertain terms that nobody loves a monomaniac and that such obsessive behavior is only going to alienate people. This won't be easy for you to do, especially since you're so full of sympathy and love. But unless somebody delivers the truth, your wife is going to have a blighted life, always feeling—and behaving—more like a walking case of diabetes than a human being with infinite interests and infinite possibilities who just happens to have diabetes.

How can I tell if a diabetic person has low blood sugar?

It helps if you know the person well enough to recognize behavior that isn't normal. If a generally easygoing person starts snapping and snarling, it may be low blood sugar. If a decisive person becomes vague, that can be a clue. Fumbling hands, glassy eyes, slurred speech, perspiration on the forehead or upper lip, a dopey smile, an odd, taut look about the face—all can be symptoms of hypoglycemia. Just about all diabetics have some signs peculiar to themselves that you'll grow to recognize if you're around them a lot and are observant.

Even if you know the person well, though, it's not always easy to recognize low blood sugar. We still remember the time we were talking to the Glendale chapter of the Diabetes Association of Southern California and told about one of our editors who said she could always recognize when June had low blood sugar "because she starts being mean to Barbara." We noticed a woman in the audience frowning. During the question-and-answer period she said, "My little boy has diabetes and takes insulin. Often, in fact, *very* often before dinner he's a holy terror. I can't do a thing with him. Could that be low blood sugar?"

"Oh boy, could it!" we chorused.

She was really shaken, because she had been punishing him for what was likely a misbehavior of his chemicals.

When you ascertain that a diabetic person does have low blood sugar, take action immediately (see page 142). Above all, don't follow the example of the sister of a diabetic friend of ours, who, when she saw he was starting to act funny, looked terrified and announced, "You've got low blood sugar! I'm getting out of here!" And she fled.

How can I keep from getting mad at my roommate when he's obnoxious because his blood sugar is low?

It's tough not to get mad. You're human, too, and sometimes you have a visceral reaction that you can't control. Just do your best to keep calm enough to help your roommate get out of the reaction, even if he fights you on it.

After the incident is over you'll probably both laugh about it. Once June had low blood sugar and became furious because she thought Barbara had eaten her dish of strawberries (which she had actually eaten herself, but couldn't remember). After her anger came despair, as she wept over her disappointment about the strawberries she had so looked forward to. With a baleful look at Barbara, she kept wailing, "You stole my strawberries." Throughout all this wrath and woe, she steadfastly refused to eat anything else to bring up her blood sugar because "the only thing I wanted was those strawberries and you ate them." In retrospect, the incident seems funny to us, but while it was going on it was like a scene out of Eugene O'Neill. At such times you feel you're dealing with an insane person. (Of course, you are.) So never take seriously or bear a grudge over something a diabetic person says or does when in hypoglycemia.

You have one big advantage in this situation: You know what low blood sugar is and can usually recognize it. This puts you way ahead of the average person. Think how people who know nothing about diabetes must react when confronted by your roommate's obnoxious behavior.

I don't like to be impatient with all the things my wife has to do to take care of her diabetes, but I admit that sometimes I am. Is there anything I can do about it?

All of us with diabetic friends or family members want them to take good care of themselves and stay healthy so we'll enjoy their love and companionship for years. And we know that taking care of diabetes takes time—lots of it. We know this intellectually but not always emotionally. For example, sometimes we're ready to go out to dinner or a movie or a sports event, and we have to stop and wait for a blood-sugar test or a snack or some diabetic something-or-other. We may get impatient, even irritated. We're not upset with the diabetic *person*, of course. It's the diabetic *condition* that bugs us. Still, the diabetic person is receiving a negative message, even if it's being delivered in a silent language.

You don't like yourself for your impatience with diabetes routines, but you can't help it. Or can you? It's possible for you to turn these moments of time that diabetes steals from you into moments that you steal for yourself. All you have to do is figure out some things you really want to do, and reserve these stolen moments to do them. You can read a book. You can work a crossword puzzle. You can play a musical instrument. You can do needlework. You can meditate. You can practice magic tricks. You can do anything that doesn't take a lot of time to set up.

If you get in the habit of truly enjoying the diabetic-routine time, it will help both you and your wife be happy. You may even start hearing yourself say to her, "Are you sure you don't want to test your blood sugar before we go out?"

What am I likely to do that will irritate my diabetic husband most?

Remember the old Paul Simon song, "Fifty Ways to Leave Your Lover"? Well, there must be 150 ways to irritate your diabetic husband. In fact, if your husband is an insulin-taker and gets low blood sugar, anything you do, including trying to get him to eat something to raise his blood sugar, is likely to bring on anything from irritation to a full-blown rage. (Some diabetic people in the throes of low blood sugar have even been known to hurl food into the face of the person trying to help.)

All persons with diabetes, even when their blood sugar is normal and even if they don't take insulin, have their pet peeves. You'll just have to find out with experience what they are.

We can start you off with a few tips, though. A diabetic person hates to hear the same phrase over and over from you. For example: "Is that on your diet?" "Did you remember to take your injection?" "Did you bring along a snack?" Anything you keep repeating begins to grate after a while.

June, for some reason, gets furious when asked, "Do you have low blood sugar?" (She claims Barbara always asks this in an accusatory tone.) Her response is usually a garbled conglomeration of "How should I know?" "Do you see a blood-sugar sensor sticking into me that I can read?" "Do you want me to stop what I'm doing and take my blood sugar; is *that* what you're saying?" Rant. Rant. Rant. She actually prefers to be told, "You're acting weird" or asked, "Why are you being so obnoxious?" probably because it's not the oft-repeated phrase that she's come to loathe.

Nagging, which one psychologist defines as "trying to control with criticism," is also near the top of the diabetic irritation scale. Nagging is not only irritating but futile. As we've repeatedly pointed out, changes are only going to be made when the diabetic person wants to make them. The best you can do is help him truly accept diabetes and to find the motivation to make the necessary changes. (See p. 36, "How do I start making all the changes I have to for my diabetes?")

Another thing that will bother your diabetic husband is your cadging snacks. Insulin takers need to carry sweets and other foods at all times in case of a reaction. If those who are aware of this rich storehouse of goodies, persist, like Goldilocks, in eating them all up, the diabetic person can be in deep trouble in an emergency when, like Old Mother Hubbard's, the snack cupboard is bare.

A far, far better thing to do is find out what your husband likes for low-blood sugar snacks and carry those yourself for diabetic emergencies—and for your own snacking pleasure.

But probably the number-one irritant for diabetic people is a lack of effort on the part of intimates to understand diabetes. Among June's close friends are some she's known for years and in whose homes she's frequently had meals. They have supposedly read most of our books, and yet they still have only a vague idea of what she can and cannot eat. They understand little about how her meals must be scheduled or what to give her when she has low blood sugar. Since these friends are not stupid, she can only infer that they don't really care. A feeling that your friends don't care goes deeper than irritation. It goes into the hurtful-wound area.

If I mention my friend's diabetes in a restaurant to try to get her something special, like a substitute for sweet-and-sour pork in a Chinese dish, she gets furious and says I make her feel like a freak. What can I do?

The answer is simplicity itself. You say to the waiter, "I am a diabetic and I can't eat anything with sugar in it. Could we please substitute pork with Chinese greens for the sweet-and-sour pork?" By claiming to be the diabetic yourself, you take the burden of asking for special favors off your friend's conscience, or pride, or whatever area of her pyschological being is disturbed.

After you've claimed to be the diabetic for a while, maybe your friend will awaken to the fact that having diabetes is nothing to be ashamed of. She will come to realize that for the most part, people in restaurants as well as in other walks of life are usually happy to help out with little problems associated with diabetes. This is an important step in her acceptance of the disease.

What should I do if we're out dining in a restaurant and my brother, who is diabetic, orders all the wrong things?

People with diabetes sometimes perversely do this. Even June, who is the most careful and rational of beings, has occasionally suffered this restaurant aberration.

The best thing to do when you hear the diabetically inappropriate meal being ordered is *not* to screech and rant and embarrass your brother in front of the waiter, but rather to order a diabetic backup meal for yourself. Very likely, when the meal is presented to him, he will take one look at it and come to his senses. Then you just say casually, without any lectures or recriminations, "It looks as if my dinner might be better for you than yours. Would you like to trade?" He probably will, with gratitude, as much gratitude for the freedom from lectures and recriminations as for the food itself.

Naturally, to perform this little sleight-of-plate act, you have to know what a diabetically appropriate meal is. So read the diet section of this book, beginning on page 40.

How do I plan a meal for my diabetic mother-in-law?

Just remember that she has to stay away from concentrated sweets— sugar, honey, and molasses in or on foods, and canned fruit in sweet syrup. Many people also have to restrict the amount of fat they eat. Ask her. Remember also that those who take insulin need a specific amount of carbohydrate in their diet. Just have something like bread, rice, pasta, or potatoes available, and she will know how much of it to eat.

That's another point to remember. Just as important as what is allowed is how much. People with diabetes must eat limited quantities of food. Don't be offended if your mother-in-law eats with gusto and then suddenly stops, as if someone has blown a whistle. There isn't a bug in the food or anything. It's just that she has eaten all that's allowed. Don't urge her to have more. That's being cruel. She would probably love to eat more, and it's taking every ounce of willpower to stop.

A basic diabetic meal would be something like this: a mixed green salad; chicken or fish or meat; potatoes or bread or pasta or rice; a vegetable or two; and fruit for dessert (either fresh or canned without sugar). Now, on the surface this may sound pretty bland, but any and all of these elements can be combined in something like beef stroganoff or bouillabaisse or chicken marengo or lamb curry. Just remember, generally, what ingredients you put into the dish and tell your mother-in-law she can estimate portions. As for drinks, read the information on alcohol (see page 68). If you're still confused about anything on the diabetic diet, just follow the advice of all the sex-manual writers who say, "If in doubt about what will be pleasing, *ask!*"

If your mother-in-law is on insulin (ask!), you should indicate at what time you're serving. This doesn't mean what time the guests are arriving but what time you'll actually have everybody sitting at the table with food on their plates. Then, once you've set the time, *stick to that time,* no matter who hasn't arrived by then (unless, of course, she's the one who's late).

Should I give up eating pastries so my diabetic sister won't feel tempted?

Admittedly, it's a little hard to sit there and wolf down a huge slab of banana cream pie if your sister is watching you like a spaniel. You both feel sorry for her, you feel guilty, and these are very digestion-upsetting emotions. Still, you definitely shouldn't give up your pastries for your sister's sake. She is going to have to get used to being tempted and resisting temptation. It's similar to the situation faced by alcoholics: they have to be able to go to a place where others are drinking and yet not drink themselves.

There remains, however, a question you didn't ask. And that is, Should you give up pastries for your own sake? Pastries are hardly the nutritional dream dish for anybody, diabetic or not. Your sister may guide you to good health and good looks.

My son wants to play football. Is that safe for a diabetic person?

There have been several outstanding diabetic football players. Ron Mix of the University of Southern California and Coley O'Brien of Notre Dame are just two. Many high-school football players shared their experiences with us when we were writing our previous books. No diabetic evil ever befell them because of football. If your son's diabetes is without complications and under good control and his doctor doesn't disapprove, then there is no reason he shouldn't play.

There are two good reasons he should. Participation in sports, especially a physically demanding one like football, will encourage him to take superb care of himself and his disease. For a young person, the incentive to keep in shape for football is far more powerful than a general incentive to watch one's health. Once your son has established good habits during his football-playing days, there's a fair chance he'll stick with them throughout his life.

He should be allowed to play football for psychological reasons as well. If his diabetes keeps him from playing football, he'll get the idea that because of diabetes he can't do anything.

On the other hand, if he plays football, his attitude will more likely be that, despite his diabetes, he can do everything he really wants to. Which attitude would you prefer him to carry through life?

Be sure he informs the coach and his teammates that he has diabetes and explains to them what they should do in case he has an insulin reaction.

And finally, do your best not to show excessive concern every time he goes out to play, even if you feel it way down inside your own pancreas. If you load him up with fears and negative feelings, you'll wreck his game and maybe cause an accident rather than prevent one. A football player needs a positive attitude above all else, and so does a diabetic.

Note: One case in which we feel you're justified in forbidding your son to play football is if your family doesn't believe in the violence of the sport and none of your children is allowed to play it. In that case it would be wrong to bend over backward and let your diabetic son do something you don't let the others do.

Should I give my brother his insulin injections?

Yes and no. Yes, you should give them to him sometimes. You can reach injection sites he can't reach himself, unless he's a contortionist. This is a big help.

Another reason for giving him his insulin is that you'll know how to give an injection. Should he ever pass out in insulin shock, you'll know how to give him glucagon (see page 187), which is injected in the same way as insulin, and bring him out of it.

But no, you shouldn't *always* give him his injection. He's got to be mainly responsible for his own insulin shooting. No one should

be that dependent on another person. It's almost like being dependent on another person for your breathing. It's not good for him or
for you, either.

What's the best way to celebrate my diabetic partner's birthday or other special occasion?

It takes some ingenuity and foresight to create the kind of birthday
celebration that's best for a person with diabetes. Fortunately, there
are now sugar-free baking and frosting mixes available. If you keep
those on hand, you'll always be ready to make something for birthday parties and other special occasions. Check with the local bakeries. As part of the diabeticization of America that we've been
talking about, many bakeries are adding sugar-free cakes to their re-
pertoires. (We know of four in the Los Angeles area.) You can even
be truly original and make something like a sandwich cake. It looks
like a cake, but when you cut into it, it's actually a club sandwich
frosted with something like blended cottage cheese and yogurt.

When it comes to gifts for diabetics, you should heed the excellent advice given in the journal *Diabetes Self-Management,* by Charles
Mallory, a Kansas City free-lance writer who has a diabetic wife:

> Don't make every gift related to diabetes. Treats don't always have to
> be sugar-free candy or dietetic chocolates, nor does a Christmas gift
> have to be a health-club membership or dinner out at the new low-
> calorie restaurant. Your wife probably likes flowers, traveling, clothes,
> and entertaining. Your husband may like cufflinks, cologne, or a
> greeting card for a special occasion. None of these has to do with dia-
> betes. Wouldn't you be disappointed if, at a birthday party, your
> friends who knew you were Catholic gave you nothing but Virgin
> Mary statuettes and rosary beads?

What should I do if I were to find a diabetic person unconscious?

Unconsciousness can be due to either diabetic coma, which means
the person has extremely high blood sugar, or insulin shock, which
means it's extremely low. If you know that person takes insulin and

sticks to his or her diet pretty well, then you can be almost certain it's insulin shock.

First, never under any circumstances pour any liquid like fruit juice or Coca-Cola down an unconscious person's throat, as it could wind up in his or her lungs and cause suffocation. The only thing you can do, if you've had good instruction and know where it is, is give an injection of glucagon. Otherwise, call the paramedics or a doctor. A word to the thrifty: an injection of glucagon costs about $40; calling the paramedics can cost over $400.

If you know for sure that the person doesn't take insulin and/or doesn't follow the diet or take care of him or herself, then it's probably a diabetic coma, the result of poor diabetes control over a long period. In this case, call the doctor or an ambulance immediately. There's nothing much you can do in this kind of crisis. Only a hospital can help now.

If you have no idea whether you're dealing with insulin shock or diabetic coma, treat for insulin shock. If it's diabetic coma, the person already has so much sugar floating throughout his or her system that a little more isn't going to make all that much difference. And if it *is* insulin shock, your quick treatment could be a lifesaver. A person in good health will eventually come out of insulin shock spontaneously, but for someone with a heart condition the shock could be life threatening.

How to Win at Losing: A Lighthearted Guide to a Lighter Body

··

The question back in the Type II section was, "How can I lose weight quickly, easily, and permanently?" The answer is you can't. But then you already knew that, didn't you? If it were possible to lose weight quickly, easily, and permanently, you wouldn't have a weight problem and neither would the 40 percent of the people over the age of forty in the United States who are classified as overweight.

Weight loss—if it is accomplished at all—comes slowly and with difficulty, and you're always at risk of putting the weight back on again.

But that doesn't mean you can't do it. You can. After all, you have that great motivator, diabetes, on your side. You want to lose weight to help keep your diabetes in control and avoid, or at least, postpone having to take insulin. That should give you more incentive than just reasons of general good health or vanity. But don't discount vanity as a motivator for losing weight. The desire to look good is right up there with the desire to feel good. Snap up any reason you can to make yourself truly effective at losing weight.

LOOKING GOOD/FEELING GOOD

Let's discuss vanity for a minute. If your idea of looking good is to be like one of those gaunt, six-foot-tall models who weigh slightly over 100 pounds that you see in women's fashion magazines or a lean but muscular surfer you see in men's sports publications, you need to readjust your thinking. You also need to accept yourself and your own body type. No matter what you do, up to and including virtual starvation, you're never going to look like that. Those thrifty genes we were talking about in the Type II section just won't let that happen.

Your more realistic goal should be to feel good and have good blood sugar, cholesterol, and triglyceride levels, and it will follow as the sunrise follows the night that you'll look good, too—and yet you'll still look like you and not like some unnatural creature from the deep world of advertising.

WEIGHT-LOSS PROGRAMS, CRASH DIETS, CELEBRITY DIETS, STRANGE DIETS

Let's say you have the desire to lose some weight to achieve the worthy health goals mentioned above. How do you go about it? As you may have noticed, there are plenty of people who are just itching—especially in the palm area—to help you. They'll guarantee to do it FAST. That's where you have to be careful. The faster the weight comes off using some kind of "fast and easy and delightful" diet or program, the more likely it is to come back again. A crash diet inevitably and invariably crashes. Those wonderful thrifty genes of yours think you're in some kind of dangerous starvation situation, so they start protecting you even more than usual, slowing down your metabolism to a snail crawl. That's why after a rigorous diet period usually even more weight comes back on than you lost. If you keep doing this yo-yo dieting over and over, it's worse for your health than to just leave on the original pounds.

Magazines that have to fill up their pages with something frequently fill them with ideas for losing weight. Favorite ones are those that caused celebrities to lose X pounds, such as "Famous Chronically Overweight Star's Secret Like Magic Wonderful Diet." No matter that in the next issue there's an article on how the same celebrity put the pounds back on again and it's either threatening her marriage or else causing her to realize that weight is not important: "It's your kind heart and what you do for others that counts." Then there are the eat-all-you-want-as-long-as-you-_____ diets. (Fill in the blank with something weird like "drink a quart of vinegar before breakfast" or "eat standing on one foot" or "eat only foods of the same color.")

But if you have a taste for different ways to lose weight, we have a few for you: some unconventional ones we've originated ourselves; others somewhat less far-out that we've gleaned from the theories of legitimate weight-loss experts. But all these ideas have at least a kernel of truth in them, and if you can incorporate a few of them into a sensible, sound weight-loss program you design for yourself, why not do it?

FALL IN LOVE

Falling in love is a great idea. An intense emotional experience could take your mind off food and at the same time instill you with the desire to be attractive to the loved one. (But it's probably even harder to run out and find someone to fall in love with than it is to lose weight in a more conventional albeit more boring way.) A cynical friend of ours suggests the opposite: "Get a divorce." But we prefer the more romantic and positive approach.

CHEW YOUR FOOD THIRTY-TWO TIMES

This is based on a theory by Horace Fletcher, a nineteenth-century nutritionist who believed you should chew food that number of times for the logical reason that we have thirty-two teeth. You hardly need to chew *that* much, but chewing food thoroughly rather than gulping it down slows the eating process. When you eat more slowly, it gives your "appestat" time to signal you that you're no longer hungry and it's time to stop eating. (Note: The dictionary defines appestat as "a presumed region in the brain, possibly in the hypothalamus, that functions to adjust appetite.") When the appestat speaks, you should listen and take its advice.

But since counting the number of chews might make you a distracted dinner companion, another way to slow your eating is to put down your fork or spoon between bites and pause a few beats before you pick it up again. Interesting dinner-table conversation can help, too, since you will want to participate, but not talk with your mouth full.

GET HAPPY

To hearken back to the first section of this book (pages 38–39), if you make yourself happy, that can help you lose weight. Contrary to the old idea that fat people are happy, it more often is unhappiness and a feeling of emotional emptiness that sends people running to the refrigerator for solace.

JUST EAT

When you eat, do nothing but eat. Of course you can engage in some delightful dinner-table conversation as suggested above or listen to some soothing background music, but don't read or watch television or do a crossword puzzle, because if you're not paying attention to your food, there's a tendency to unconsciously shovel it in. On top of that, you hardly taste what you're eating and don't enjoy your meal very much. Above all, dining should be pleasurable. We've noticed that the better tasting and more enjoyable food is, the sooner you feel fully satisfied and the less you tend to eat.

EAT IN ONE PLACE

Eat only in a designated eating place—in your dining room or on the kitchen table or at the breakfast bar. That way you don't wander around the house snacking all the time. And you certainly don't snack sitting in front of the television or in a moving car. Not that we're knocking snacks as such. Nancy Cooper, R.D., in her book *The Joy of Snacks,* says that for people with Type II diabetes, "snacks provide a way to distribute calories evenly during the day to help the body's insulin work better and keep blood glucose (sugar) levels more stable. Eating smaller meals with between-meal snacks also helps people with diabetes control their appetites and may make weight loss easier." The only problem would be if you eat a bunch of snacks on top of normal-size meals at breakfast, lunch, and dinner. But even if you're on a small meal and snack program, you still should eat everything in a designated eating place.

WRITE IT DOWN

Another sound suggestion is to write down everything you eat—and we do mean everything, right down to the breath mint you might have after lunch. Seeing there in black and white everything you've eaten and the approximate number of calories it contains can vividly show you where you're going wrong and where those unwanted pounds are coming from. It also gets pretty tedious writing all that stuff down, so conceivably you'll start deciding to skip eating something in order to avoid having to get out your notebook and record it.

Keeping a careful record of what you eat can be very effective in a weight-loss program. A University of Pittsburgh School of Medicine study showed that people with Type II diabetes on a weight-loss program who meticulously recorded what they ate lost an average of thirty-seven pounds, whereas those who wrote in a haphazard and irregular way lost an average of only ten pounds.

BRUSH YOUR TEETH

Here's an idea that will make for good dental health as well as weight loss. Any time you eat anything, brush and floss your teeth thoroughly. Just like writing down everything you eat, this will soon become so boring and time-consuming that you'll often decide it's not worth it and skip the food.

EAT ONLY WHEN YOU'RE HUNGRY

On the surface this may seem ridiculous. Why else would you eat? Well, many of us eat for lots of other reasons: because we're bored, because we're nervous, because we're depressed, because we're tired, because we're trying to be polite, and even for the Mount Everest reason, because the food is there. Let your body rather than your emotions tell you when it's time to eat.

But we realize that in your case eating when you're hungry can be a problem. People with Type II diabetes can be hungry most of the time because of the excess quantities of insulin floating around in their bloodstreams. At times you may even move from the realm of hunger into being totally, almost uncontrollably ravenous. We received a letter from one woman who asked plaintively, "How do I get past my horrible cravings for chocolate, sweet donuts, etc., just before my monthly period?"

For the answer to that we turned to Virginia Valentine, a Type II herself, and one who, through the courtesy of excess insulin has often felt so hungry she could, as she says, "eat a whole wheat-field." Her advice is not to fight your cravings, but to give in to them. A deprivation mind-set often brings on bingeing. You definitely don't want that to happen to you. What you must do, she advises, is "creative munching." Find things you can eat that will satisfy your cravings but not blow your weight control and your diabetes control out of the water.

Her suggestions include low-sugar, low-fat frozen chocolate yogurt; strawberries dipped into Wax Orchards Fudge Sweet, a delicious dark fudge sauce that is virtually fat free and made with a fruit concentrate. (Available from SugarFree Centers, 1-800-323-7221 or directly from Wax Orchards, 1-800-634-6132.)

Fudge Sweet is also wonderful on fat-free ice cream (which is not all that tasty by itself) and put between vanilla wafers to make a kind of "reverse Oreo." Chocolate Cool Whip is another enlivener of ice cream and makes a great parfait when you layer it with sugar-free pudding. You can take Virginia's ideas and build on them with your own favorites, but just make sure they are as low-sugar and low-fat as hers.

BREAKFAST LIKE A KING, LUNCH LIKE A PRINCE, DINNER LIKE A PAUPER

For your diabetes control it would be best to distribute your daily intake of calories exactly equally between the three meals. Not easy to do. For weight loss, it would be best to have your largest meal at breakfast, a medium-size meal at lunch, and the smallest meal at dinner. This is because your metabolism (rate at which you burn calories) slows down at night and you tend to store more of what you eat then.

But we have to be realistic. A meal plan like that wouldn't work too well in our society—and possibly in your family—so you'll have to make some adjustments to reality. You can lose weight with a *moderate* breakfast (never skip breakfast!), lunch, and dinner. If you're eating out and have a choice of when you go, you're much better off making it lunch rather than dinner. For one thing, the portions they serve at lunch are usually smaller, and for another, it's usually much less expensive.

If you must, for career, social, psychological, or familial reasons eat your largest meal at night, then eat as early as you can, preferably no later than 6:00. (And eat nothing after dinner. No snacks allowed, unless, of course, you take insulin and have a bout of low blood sugar.) When we go to New York, for example, we always try to have lunch (a fixed price one if possible) at a nice restaurant.

Then we eat a light supper, maybe just a sandwich and salad, or else a "pre-theater supper." These are, like lunch, smaller and less expensive and you have to eat early to get them. The prices and portions go up dramatically at 6:30 or 7:00.

FEED YOUR DOGGIE BAG

Dining out in the evening the portions are often huge. We solve this by taking about half the protein serving (and sometimes some of the peripherals as well) home for lunch or dinner the next day. People who feel they might succumb to the temptation to eat everything they're served if it's there on the plate tell us that they ask for the doggie bag when the meal is served and put half of the food out of harm's way before they even lift a fork.

AVOID BUFFETS

Here's a statistic that may serve to drive you from the buffet groaning boards. The average person eats 2.5 pounds of food at a buffet, but only 1.2 pounds at a sit-down meal. Think what that could do to a person with an insulin-driven appetite! Type I's and Type II's who have a natural tendency to be thin, like June, may have the opposite reaction. When she's faced with a huge buffet display, it scares her appetite away because she thinks all that food is sure to send her blood sugar sky-high. Consequently, she pulls back on her eating so much that she usually winds up with low blood sugar and has to take glucose tablets to bring it up.

A LICENSE TO LOSE WEIGHT

Virginia Valentine came up with another good idea recently. (She has a lot of them!) Her daughter was taking out her first driver's license and brought it home to show her mother. "Melanie, what have you done?" she said. "You put down your real weight." Melanie was baffled. "Of course I did. What else would I put down?"

"What you should do is put down the weight you want to be," explained Virginia. "That way every time you look at your license and see that weight, it's an inspiration—almost a religious experience."

You do have to be a little realistic—don't knock off fifty pounds—but shaving your weight a little can keep the goal constantly in mind until you make it come true.

THE BASIC TWO

Up to now we've been dealing pretty much with the psychology of weight loss and have given you some little tricks of the trade to help you manage your food and your hunger better. But now we're coming to the meat and potatoes—so to speak—of losing pounds. Without these two, all the tricks above won't work. With these two and a few of the tricks above, you can't fail.

EAT LESS FAT

A nondiabetic friend who has a chronic weight problem picked up one useful morsel of information in one of the many expensive weight-loss programs she attended: fat makes you fat. It's that simple and that true. Fat of all kinds—the so-called "good" fats, the monounsaturated and polyunsaturated kind, and the "bad" fats, the saturated vegetable and animal fats—are all equally bad as far as fat-making is concerned. The sad fact of the matter is that a gram of fat contains 9 calories while a gram of protein or carbohydrate contains only 4. It doesn't take a mathematical wizard to see the difference and what to avoid if you want to lose or control weight. Fat also can pop right into the old fat cells without being processed.

Therefore they burn fewer calories than carbohydrates and proteins do in the processing process. Some people have peeled off pounds by the simple expedient of avoiding fats. Fat avoidance is one of the cornerstones of the well-known Pritikin weight-loss program.

Besides putting on and keeping on weight, fat is bad for you in other ways, implicated as it is in cardiovascular disease, some forms of cancer, gallbladder disease, and joint problems. Then consider the problems it causes for your diabetes. The physical stress of carrying around extra weight brings out your genetic tendency to develop diabetes and raises blood sugar after you develop it because that same fat makes your cells even more insulin-resistant than they already are.

Just how much fat should you have in your diet? The question would be better put, how *little* fat? Debra Waterhouse, M.P.H., R.D., author of the excellent book *Outsmarting the Female Fat Cell*, says that 20 percent is a realistic figure that is "low enough to significantly reduce your risk of heart disease and cancer—and reduce your weight." She thinks that if you could reduce fat to 10 percent, it would be even better, but that going that low "may cause feelings of restriction and deprivation." (Remember what Virginia Valentine says happens if you feel too deprived!)

To bring that percentage figure into dietary reality, you take your total daily allotment of calories and multiply by 20 percent. That gives you your number of allowable calories of fat. Then divide that by 9 to give you the number of grams of fat you can have. You can fill in the blanks to make a chart for yourself.

Total calories per day = _____
$\times$ 20% (.20) = _____
$\div$ 9 = _____ grams of fat per day

We once heard Julia Child speak to a group of dietitians and tell them she wished they would stop talking about grams because Americans just don't understand them. But it's important to think grams these days because the new packaging laws are going to tell you the contents of products in terms of grams.

Fat by the Gram

When you look at a package, while not ignoring the sugar content, focus most carefully on the grams of fat. Now, we're not saying that you should never eat any product or food item that is over 20 percent fat. That would leave out having even small amounts of butter or margarine or olive oil. No, you just have to balance it all out. If you have some things that are over 20 percent fat, you can lower the percentage of fat in your diet by including others that are only 10 percent or 5 percent or no fat at all. And remember—Julia Child notwithstanding—if you deal in grams, all you have to remember is the total number of grams of fat you're allowed per day and stay within that range whatever individual foods you're eating.

It's not always easy to know how many grams of fat you're eating. Fat lurks everywhere, and you have to be a fat detective to find it. To do this, you will need a book like *The Fat Counter,* by Annette B. Natow and Jo-Ann Heslin. (There are many other similar books now available. Look for those that include, along with the basics, packaged and frozen foods, prepared mixes, snacks, and food from fast-food chains.) When you get your fat guide, read it like a novel all the way through and keep it handy, like a Bible, for constant reference and inspiration. In these books you'll find many surprises. We know we did. For example, we'd always heard that flank steak was the leanest cut of beef you can get, so on the few times that we eat beef, we would always select that, although we might prefer some other cut, especially Barbara, who likes a steak with a bone to gnaw on. On reading *The Fat Counter* we discovered that what we'd heard was not always true. 3 oz. of broiled flank steak contain 11 grams of fat, while if you eat 3 oz. of the lean part of a T-bone, that's only 9 grams. So you see, knowing the fat content of foods can also sometimes allow you to eat what you really want over something you think would be better for you.

FAT PITFALLS

There are pitfalls in your path of fat avoidance. Some you should especially try to sidestep include:

The Great Salad Fallacy

People often think they're having a low-calorie lunch when they have "just a salad," and so they are—until the salad dressing is plopped or drizzled all over it. This can turn a 100-calorie salad with no fat into a 500-calorie monster, 360 of which calories are fat. Always, *always* order your dressing on the side. Another trick is to not put that on-the-side dressing on the salad, but just dip your fork into it before you spear your lettuce and other salad ingredients. That way you'll get enough dressing to taste but not enough to do harm. Warning: if the dressing is something gloppy like a thick bleu cheese or Roquefort, dip your fork into it with the tines facing straight down and shake off the excess. If you scoop a thick dressing up, a fork can carry almost as much as a spoon and that will destroy the whole fork-dip theory.

Incidentally, a safe and tasty salad dressing is salsa, which is appearing on more and more restaurant tables these days. (Salsa sales have now overtaken the sales of catsup.) Since salsa has little or no fat, only tomatoes, onions, peppers, and seasonings, you can feel free to use more of that.

Another salad fallacy is that since you've eaten only a salad, you "can handle" and you "deserve" a nice, rich, sweet dessert. Need we say how false this fallacy is?

The Great Bran Muffin Fallacy

Often when you're having a coffee break at a cafe or restaurant or bakery and you look around and see the array of cinnamon rolls and Danish pastries, foods you know are full of sugar and fat, you may sigh with relief when you spot a bran muffin. "Ah, at least there's *one thing* here that's healthy. I'll have a bran muffin, please."

Morton H. Shaevitz, Ph.D., author of the insightful and innovative *Lean & Mean: The No-Hassle, Life-Extending Weight Loss Program for Men,* sets us straight on that one. He calls a commercial bran muffin "a fat sponge." It's particularly sad when you're trying really hard to do the right thing—such as choose the bran muffin—and it turns out to be one of the most wrong things you can do. But bran muffins are not forever denied you. You can make delicious healthy ones yourself. This is June's favorite bran muffin recipe. She assembles the dry ingredients the night before so that even if she's a little groggy in the morning, she can quickly and easily whip up a batch for breakfast.

June's "Health Sponge" Bran Muffins

1 cup whole wheat flour	2 tbsp. Fruit Sweet*
3 tsp. baking powder	1 egg
½ tsp. salt (optional)	1 cup nonfat milk
1 cup bran	raisins (optional)
2 tbsp. vegetable oil	

*Fruit Sweet is a fruit concentrate sweetener available from Wax Orchards, 1-800-634-6132.

Preheat the oven to 425°. Sift together flour, baking powder, and salt (optional). Add bran and stir thoroughly. In a separate, smaller bowl, mix together vegetable oil, Fruit Sweet, the egg, and milk. Add this mixture to the dry ingredients and mix only enough to moisten. Fill Pam-sprayed muffin tins or tins lined with paper baking cups (you can also spray these), ⅔ full. Bake for 15 minutes or until done. As a variation you can add the raisins either to the whole batch or to half of it.

8 servings   Exchanges per serving: 1 starch; 1 fat   Calories: 142
Protein: 6 gm   Carbohydrate: 23 gm   Fat: 5 gm
Fiber: 4 gm   Cholesterol: 27 mg   Sodium: 268 mg

Cocktail Hour Snacks

Who knows how many grams of fat lurk in cocktail hour snacks? Hardly anybody knows because there are too many to even comprehend. Oh, the nuts! Oh, the chips! Oh, the dips! Oh, the cheese-laden goodies! Oh, the cocktail sausages! Oh, we could go on and on, but you get the drift. You could consume way more than your whole day's ration of fat in an hour at the cocktail party. See if you can find any pretzels. They are the least harmful (except for the salt). See if someone with dietary intelligence has put out carrot or celery sticks or radishes. (Don't dip them in the dressing that is undoubtedly provided.) If you don't see anything that a person who isn't there to lap up fat would go for, then turn your back on the table. (Get thee behind me!)

While we're discussing cocktail snacks, we might as well mention what goes with the cocktail snacks—**alcohol.** Alcohol has seven calories per gram, almost as many as fat, so when you drink a cocktail you could think of the alcohol in it as "liquid fat." (Yum!)

If you're in a serious weight-loss program, you might heed the advice of non-muffin man Morton H. Shaevitz: "While you're trying to lose weight, drink no alcohol at all." After you've reached the weight you want to be, then "limit yourself to two drinks a day," which is good advice for everyone diabetic or not, overweight or not.

Drinking alcohol during the cocktail hour carries the additional risk of possibly lowering your inhibitions and increasing your hunger to the extent that you dive into those forbidden snacks. If you're going to drink something alcoholic during the course of the evening, you might be better off just having club soda (with a twist and maybe a dash of bitters) or a diet soft drink (with a squirt of lime) during the cocktail hour and then enjoy a glass of good wine with your dinner.

Movie Snacks

Years ago a movie marketing genius figured out they could make more money on the snacks than on the tickets, so the food counter in theaters grew and grew until it has reached the outlandish proportions of today. They've also extended the intermissions so you'll have more than plenty of time to line up and buy. It gets boring waiting for the almost interminable intermission to be over, and when you see everyone else chomping away on buttery popcorn and ice cream bars and candy and, in some cases, even hot dogs, the temptation to join the ravening crowd can be almost overwhelming.

One alternative we suggest is smuggling in your own fat-free, air-popped popcorn. Popcorn is an ideal high-fiber snack, filling and low calorie. If you're subtle enough, no one will notice what you're doing, and if you want to add a sugar-free soda from the Great Temptation Counter in the lobby, then you can be just as happy and satisfied as anyone in the theater—and make just as much noise and mess.

Stand-ins for Fat

Now, when you cut all of that fat out of your diet, you're going to have to replace it with *something.* Animal proteins usually contain a goodly (or badly!) portion of fat—and fat of the least desirable saturated kind—so you'll need to go light on them, cutting off all visible fat on meat and removing the skin from poultry. (That's where the fat is deposited.) Eating fish is another good option. You can also turn to plentiful, inexpensive carbohydrates, some of which, like beans and legumes, can be combined with wheat products for a balanced vegetable protein that is extremely low in fat. It takes a bit of self-education to learn to balance vegetable protein, but many vegetarians happily and healthily do it. The book *The New Laurel's Kitchen* is particularly recommended for this, as well as for its delicious recipes. Unlike many vegetarian-cookbook writers, Laurel doesn't believe in using lots of concentrated sweets in her recipes.

In dealing with carbohydrates, what you want are the complex carbohydrates (starches) rather than simple carbohydrates (sugars). You should also select complex carbohydrates that contain a lot of fiber (grains, fruits, and vegetables) because fiber slows down the absorption of sugars and starches in the intestine and helps keep your blood sugar from raising as high or as fast after a meal. Fiber also provides bulk that will make you feel fuller with fewer calories (fiber is virtually calorie-free), so you don't feel like eating so much. Enough fiber virtually eliminates any need for laxatives in your life and helps prevent hemorrhoids and many digestive disorders. On top of that, fiber-rich foods generally have to be chewed more, so that slows down your eating. (See above.)

Incidentally, certain fibers, besides helping with your weight-loss program, also serve to lower cholesterol, thereby possibly helping prevent the cardiovascular diseases to which Type II's are susceptible. These include pectins, which are found in fruit; guar gum from beans; and the fiber in rolled oats and carrots. The best idea is to keep all your health bases covered by eating a variety of fiber-rich foods.

An excellent guide to putting more fiber of all kinds in your diet and—not incidentally—less fat is *Diabetes: A New Guide to Healthy Living,* by James W. Anderson, M.D. (see Recommended Reading). This book contains a chart of the fiber content of foods and sample diets.

Pyramid Club

One good thing the government has done lately is come up with the food pyramid. Originally called "the eating right pyramid," it shows you not just what foods you should eat as the old "basic four groups" did, but how much of each. As you can see from this and from what we've said so far, all foods are not created equal. With some more is better and with others less is imperative.

Although many food special-interest groups—we're sure you can guess which ones—tried to get the government to drop the recommendations of the pyramid or at least to modify them, it stuck to its guns just about as well as you can ever expect it to in the face of heavy lobbying, and in the end the pyramid remains fairly true to the original concept.

Food Guide Pyramid

A Guide to Daily Food Choices

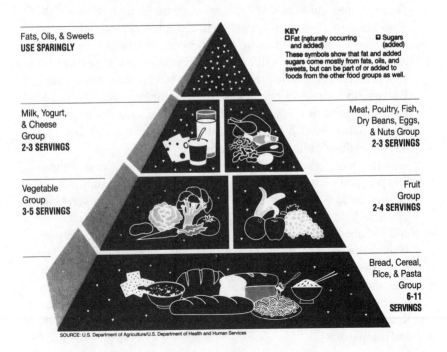

Fats, Oils, & Sweets
USE SPARINGLY

KEY
□ Fat (naturally occurring   ▪ Sugars
  and added)   (added)
These symbols show that fat and added sugars come mostly from fats, oils, and sweets, but can be part of or added to foods from the other food groups as well.

Milk, Yogurt,
& Cheese
Group
2-3 SERVINGS

Meat, Poultry, Fish,
Dry Beans, Eggs,
& Nuts Group
2-3 SERVINGS

Vegetable
Group
3-5 SERVINGS

Fruit
Group
2-4 SERVINGS

Bread, Cereal,
Rice, & Pasta
Group
6-11
SERVINGS

SOURCE: U.S. Department of Agriculture/U.S. Department of Health and Human Services

By the way, in the vegetable and fruit groups, be sure to eat the whole fruit and the whole vegetable. The juices don't contain enough fiber and are therefore more likely to raise your blood sugar higher and faster. Avoid them, no matter what the Juiceman may say.

Think of this pyramid sprinkled all over with fiber and you'll have just the right image to carry in your mind as you go forth to select the kind of meals that will help you to lose the weight, which will, in turn, help your diabetes.

EXERCISE MORE!

We've said it before (see pages 80–85) but we can't say it too often. Exercise is a basic part of diabetes therapy; almost a magic formula for people with diabetes. This is particularly true for Type II's.

Just look at these magic properties it has for you. It can keep you from having to take insulin by making your cells more receptive to the insulin you have, and it helps you lose weight three ways:

1. It burns up calories.

2. It fights those dratted thrifty genes of yours by enlivening your sluggish metabolism so your body uses more calories at all times, for all of its functions, including those physical and mental processes that take place even while you're sitting still or sleeping. Some people have rapid rates of metabolism—the lucky devils. These are the people who can stuff down mountains of anything they want to eat and remain as skinny as a broom handle. While exercise won't take you that far into the land of the rapid metabolism, it will take you in that direction. Changing your metabolism is the whole point behind many proven effective weight-loss programs, including Covert Bailey's *Fit or Fat* series of books and his Public Broadcasting System TV programs.

3. It suppresses your appetite so you don't feel hungry all the time. That may come as a surprise. Most people think that exercise stimulates your appetite when just the opposite is true. Perhaps mild, not-really-exercise exercise might make your stomach start to turn its thoughts toward food, but the kind of brisk, minimum of

20–30 minutes of aerobic exercise you need on an effective program shuts off the hunger machine. As one of our nutritional heroes, Dr. Jean Meyer, said, "You have three choices: you can exercise more, you can always feel hungry, or you can be fat." It's not hard to see which of these is the best choice.

But, while encouraging you with these good and true positives, although we don't like to motivate people negatively, we have to throw in one threat: *it is a virtual certainty that you won't be able to lose weight and keep it off without exercise.* That's a simple fact. Diet alone will not work for you. The more you starve yourself— and starvation is so agonizing that you can't keep it up very long— the more your body decides to get along on fewer calories in order to keep the amount it needs in its fat-saving bank to feel secure and protected.

Fighting Exercise Resistance

If even after reading the exercise pep talk on pages 80–85, you still feel you have a reason to resist exercise, let's try to shoot it down. If the reason is mental: "I just can't get motivated" or "I don't have the time to fit it in," we won't buy it. The exercise has to be enough of a priority in your life and health that you won't let self-imposed psychological barriers keep you away from it. Just grit your teeth and do it. Before long you'll find you're using those teeth for smiling at the weight-loss and the good feelings the exercise has generated.

Physical problems are another matter, although these too can usually be overcome. We asked Claudia Graham, Ph.D., M.P.H., director of the Diabetes Management Center of the Presbyterian Intercommunity Hospital in Whittier, California, for her advice on exercise for people who can't exercise. Claudia knows whereof she speaks since she is a diabetes exercise therapist as well as an avid sportsperson and, to top it all off, she has diabetes herself.

She recommends walking as the best overall exercise for people with physical problems. Mall walking is particularly good since it's companionable (there are many mall-walking clubs) and safe.

And since it's not affected by the weather, you have no excuse not to do it.

If walking is difficult and painful for you because of foot or joint problems (particularly the knee), she suggests using a stationary bicycle with toe clips at its lowest possible tension setting. That way you aren't putting any weight on your knees, and also, with very little resistance in the pedaling, you're less likely to stress them.

She also recommends water exercise, since the water supports you. Unfortunately, sometimes it supports you too much. Since fat floats, people who haven't yet lost the weight they need to may just bob around, and that doesn't burn calories or rev up your metabolism. In that case, a kickboard helps. As you propel yourself around the pool, try to kick your legs a little higher than your floating body if you can. Claudia says most YMCAs and many senior centers have pools, and those that do usually have water exercise classes. These cost only a dollar or two to attend and give you a fantastic return in safe exercise benefits.

Claudia advises people with physical problems to forget the "no pain, no gain" theory of exercise fanatics and follow instead her "If it hurts, don't do it" motto. But even if you have physical problems that limit the amount of exercise you can do, her most important piece of advice is, "Anything is better than nothing at all."

If you have any kind of physical limitations, especially a cardiovascular condition, you should by all means check with your doctor before embarking on an exercise program. Once he or she gives the green light or even a yellow one indicating proceed with caution, then the very best thing you can do for yourself is have a consultation with an exercise therapist. Your diabetes educator or a hospital in your area that specializes in diabetes should be able to recommend a therapist who understands both your diabetes and whatever other conditions you have that limit your exercise. Working with your therapist, you will find the most effective exercise that your physical condition will permit. You will surely find that your sessions with the therapist will be the best investment you can make for your weight-loss program, your diabetes, your health, and your life.

FINAL STRATEGIES

Liquid-Diet Programs

We've often been asked if those liquid diets are good for diabetic weight-loss programs. These are more for people who fall into the obese rather than the overweight category. The Mayo Clinic recommends such plans only for people who are at least fifty pounds overweight or 30 percent heavier than what would be considered their ideal weight. Even in that case, these diets should be undertaken only under the advice and careful guidance of a physician. This holds true for anybody—but especially for a person with diabetes.

Weight-Loss Support Groups

Some weight-loss support groups can be very effective as long as they are truly supportive and don't make a ritual of ridiculing people who haven't reached their week's goal of lost pounds. We've known a number of people, both diabetic and non, who achieved long-lasting success with Overeaters Anonymous. If you do find a compatible support group, it can do a lot to inspire you. Losing weight is like what has been said about dying; it's something you ultimately have to do alone, but it's a great comfort to have someone there to hold your hand while it's happening.

While you're losing your weight, think of us as holding your hand. We will be. And we won't let it go until we have to in order to applaud you for achieving your desired goal!

Reference Section

. . . .

Medications that increase blood-glucose levels

Chlorthalidone
Corticosteroids
Diazoxide
Furosemide
Epinephrine-like medications
Estrogens
Nicotinic acid
Phenytoin
Syrups containing sugar
Thyroid preparations
Thiazide
Glucagon
Caffeine (large quantities)
Cyclophosphamide
Ethacrynic acid
Asparaginase
Morphine
Nicotine
Lithium

Medications that lower blood-glucose levels

Ethyl alcohol
Insulin
Sulfonylureas
Beta blockers
Anabolic steroids
Fenfluramine
Biguanides
Salicylates (large doses)
Disopyramide
Phenobarbital (and other
    enzyme inducers)

Directory of Organizations

American Association of Diabetes Educators
444 N. Michigan Ave., Ste. 1240
Chicago, IL 60601
1-800-338-DMED
Write for information on diabetes education programs and a list of
certified diabetes educators in your area.

American Diabetes Association
1660 Duke St.
Alexandria, VA 22314
1-800-ADA-DISC
Write for the address of your local chapter if it is not listed in your
phone book.

American Dietetic Association
216 W. Jackson Blvd., Ste. 800
Chicago, IL 60606-6995
312-899-0040, ext. 5800
Can provide names of qualified dietitians in your area.

International Diabetic Athletes Association
6829 N. 12th St., Ste. 205
Phoenix, AZ 85014
602-230-8155
A nonprofit organization to foster interaction among active individuals with diabetes who participate in sports and fitness activities at
all levels, health care professionals, and everyone interested in the
relationship between (or special problems of) diabetes and sports.

Juvenile Diabetes Foundation International
432 Park Avenue South
New York, NY 10016-8103
1-800-223-1138
A national group whose objective is to fund research aimed at cur-
ing diabetes and preventing its complications. Information, educational programs, and meetings for diabetic children and young
people and their families. Write for address of your local chapter.

How Sweet It Is

Aspartame	A protein sweetener 180 times as sweet as sucrose. Technically, aspartame is caloric; however, it is so sweet that the amount used per serving of food is likely to supply almost no calories. Marketed as Equal and NutraSweet.
Carob Powder Carob flour	Produced by grinding the pod of the carob tree. Tastes similar to chocolate. Seventy-five percent is made up of sucrose, glucose, and fructose, which are all caloric.
*Cyclamates**	*Noncaloric* sweeteners approximately thirty times as sweet as sucrose. Cyclamates were banned from use in the United States in 1970 because of questions about their possible cancer- and tumor-causing properties. They are still used in some foreign countries, and the risk associated with moderate use is considered by many to be very small. In 1989 it was announced that the U.S. ban on cyclamates would be lifted, but this has not happened.
Dextrin	Chains of glucose molecules. Their effect on blood glucose has not been well evaluated but may be similar to glucose. Caloric.
Dulcitol	A sugar alcohol. Caloric.
Fructose Fruit sugar Levulose	One of the most common naturally occurring sugars, particularly found in fruit and honey. It is not associated with a rapid and high rise in blood sugar in well-controlled diabetes. The sweetness of refined fructose varies, but under certain conditions it can be almost twice as sweet as sucrose. Caloric.

*The sweeteners in italics are generally felt to be appropriate sweeteners for the diabetic individual, provided they are used according to the recommendation of a physician or dietitian.

Glucose
  Corn sugar
  Dextrose
  Grape sugar
	A naturally occurring sugar that normally causes a fast and high rise in blood sugar. About half as sweet as table sugar. Carbohydrates (starches) break down to glucose during digestion, as do all sugars eventually. Glucose is the form of sugar that the body uses for energy and other purposes, and it builds up in the blood if diabetes is poorly controlled. *Dextrose* is the commercial name for glucose and will often be seen on food labels, including those of some sugar substitutes. Caloric.

Glucose Syrups
  Corn syrup
  Corn-syrup solids
  Sorghum syrup
  Starch syrup
  Sugar-cane syrup
	Liquid sweeteners produced by the breakdown (hydrolyzation) of starch. They contain a mixture of glucose, maltose, and longer chains of glucose molecules and can be produced from a variety of starches (hence, the varied names). *Corn-syrup solids* are the crystallized form of corn syrup. Caloric.

High-Fructose Corn Syrups	Produced from corn syrups. They contain differing amounts of fructose, ranging from 42 to 90 percent. The remaining part of the syrup is primarily glucose. The effect of the highly refined type (90 percent fructose) on blood glucose has not been well evaluated, but, theoretically, it should not cause high and fast rises of glucose in the blood of people whose diabetes is well controlled. The 90 percent type is the only one that might prove to be an acceptable sweetener for diabetics. Caloric.

Honey
  Comb honey
  Creamed honey
	A natural syrup that varies in sugar and flavor depending on many factors. It is primarily glucose (about 35 percent), fructose (about 40 percent), and water and, by weight, is about 75 percent as sweet as sucrose. Additional glucose is sometimes added to some honeys. Caloric.

Lactose	Milk sugar. It comprises about 4.5 percent of cow milk. About 30 percent as sweet as sucrose. Caloric.

Maltose	Two glucose units linked together. It is only 30 to 50 percent as sweet as sucrose, but it rapidly breaks down to glucose in the intestinal tract. Caloric.
Mannitol	A naturally occurring sugar alcohol that causes less of a rise in blood sugar than do sucrose or glucose. It is about half as sweet as sucrose and is slowly absorbed into the blood. In large amounts, it can cause diarrhea. Caloric.
Maple Syrup Maple sugar	Made from the sap of the maple and other trees. It is mostly sucrose, with some invert sugar (see *sucrose*) and trace amounts of other compounds. The crystallized syrup is *maple sugar.* Caloric.
Milk Chocolate Bitter chocolate Bittersweet chocolate	Produced by the addition of milk, sugar, and cocoa butter to bitter chocolate. *Milk chocolate* is approximately 43 percent sugar and *bittersweet chocolate* is about 40 percent sugar. The sugar is caloric.
Molasses Blackstrap Golden syrup Refiners' syrup Treacle Unsulphured	The sugar drawn from sugar crystals as they are refined into pure sucrose. Different types are usually produced during sucrose refinement. All types, however, contain 50 to 75 percent sugar (sucrose and invert sugar) and should generally be avoided by diabetics. The sugars are caloric.
Saccharin	The currently used *noncaloric* sweetener in the United States. It is about 375 times as sweet as sucrose.
Sorbitol	A naturally occurring sugar alcohol found in many plants; commercially produced from glucose. It is about half as sweet and more slowly absorbed than glucose. In individuals whose diabetes is well controlled, it causes only a small postmeal rise in blood glucose. In large amounts it may cause diarrhea. It is widely used in the manufacture of dietetic foods and chewing gums. Caloric.

Sucrose
  Beet sugar
  Brown sugar
  Cane sugar
  Confectioner's
    sugar
  Invert sugar
  Powdered sugar
  Raw sugar
  Saccharose
  Sugar
  Table sugar
  Turbinado
	A naturally occurring sugar that is composed of equal parts of glucose and fructose linked together. It is produced from sugar cane or sugar beets. *Invert sugar* is made of sucrose that has been broken down to equal parts of glucose and fructose (with some sucrose left intact). *Brown sugars, raw sugar,* and *Turbinado* all contain some molasses.

Sweetened
  Condensed
    whole milk
  Sweetened
    condensed
    skim milk
  Sweetened
    condensed
    whey
	Produced by reducing the water content of milk by about half and adding sugar. The finished product is about 44 percent sucrose, which is caloric. This means a fourteen-ounce can of condensed whole milk contains the equivalent of eight tablespoons of sugar and two and a half cups of milk.

Xylitol	A naturally occurring sugar alcohol produced from xylose (bark sugar). It is slowly absorbed and causes less of a rise in blood sugar than does sucrose or glucose. Depending on how it is used, it is as sweet as or less sweet than sucrose. It is believed to be less cavity inducing than other sugars. Large amounts can cause diarrhea, and questions about its safety have held up its use in all but a few products. Caloric.

Courtesy of Phyllis Crapo, R.D., and Margaret A. Powers, R.D., *Diabetes Forecast,* March–April 1981, p. 24. Copyright 1980 by the American Diabetes Association. Reprinted from *Diabetes Forecast* with permission.

Reverend Eaton's Notice to the Hostess

Dear Hostess:

Rev. Eaton is on a special diet. I am enclosing a <u>sample</u> of his routine to help you to understand what it involves.

> NOTE: There can be <u>NO SUGAR</u> in the preparation of any of his foods.

Below is his basic diet for one day:

BREAKFAST:
>   8 ounces unsweetened juice
>   2 slices toast—16 ounces milk
>   2 eggs—1¾ cup dry cereal

LUNCH:
>   4 ounces meat (after cooked)
>   3 slices bread (or equivalent—i.e., 3 small potatoes)
>   8 ounces milk
>   2 pieces fruit (i.e., apples, pears, peaches, whole)
>   ½ cup vegetable (i.e., string beans, lettuce, asparagus, celery, tomatoes)

DINNER:
>   Same as for lunch.

BEDTIME SNACK:
>   2 slices bread—2 ounces meat
>   8 ounces milk—2 pieces fruit

THANK YOU for your willingness to entertain us, and helpfulness in this matter.

In His Service,
Mrs. G. Eaton

The Dragon Diabetes

(A Grimm Fairy Tale)
by Joan Williams Hoover

Washington, D.C., where I live, is a city where history is made, and almost anything can happen. Let me tell you about a fantasy I had in this magical kingdom:

One day I went downtown to the Smithsonian Institution and walked into the Hall of Dinosaurs, in the Natural History Museum. I stood before a great rack of bones, and listened to the docent tell me about the terrible Dragon Diabetes, who had once roamed the face of the Earth.

She told how the dragon had once grabbed innocent people, including little children and old people, and hurt them, and made their lives very difficult.

How it had tormented them while they tried to fight it off with sharpened needles.

How it snatched away their food, and some days left them weak and disoriented.

How the people never dared forget about the dragon for even a single hour, lest he sneak up behind and blast them with his fiery breath.

And how, when some of the people thought they had finally learned to live in peace with the dragon, he would suddenly lash out and blind their eyes, or bite off their legs, or cast an evil spell onto their hearts and kidneys.

Sometimes he just took these brave people off to his cave and they were never seen again.

He was a TERRIBLE dragon!

The people threw lots of money at him (in those days they believed that enough money would cure almost anything).

And they poked holes in their bodies, hoping to defy him by taking out red juice and putting in white juice.

And they invented wonderful little machines intended to keep the dragon under control (except that the machines only gave results. They never explained causes, nor provided any solutions).

And they waved their 1200 calorie diets at the dragon, and threw him great hunks of ugly fat . . . but still he raged on.

Eventually the people got so desperate that they even started to blame each other. They shook their fingers and told each other that if they had only been more careful, perhaps the dragon might not have noticed them in the first place.

Finally the people could stand the dragon no longer and they declared a war. They were determined to win. They knew they weren't bigger than the dragon, but certainly they were a lot smarter.

They looked hard at what they had been doing in years past. They had left the job to politicians, medical researchers, diabetes organizations and others, and they saw that it hadn't worked. The threat was as great as ever.

They realized that for years they had been paying experts handsomely to do little more than just throw pebbles at the dragon . . . experts who danced around claiming that they were right on the brink of doing away with the dragon . . . if only the people would send more money . . . and not ask too many questions.

Sometimes the experts would get to fighting among themselves, over things like money, or power, or recognition, and FORGET that they were there to fight the dragon.

The dragon loved that because HE never forgot. He NEVER took a day off, and he NEVER slept.

Finally, all the people got together. They thought and thought. Soon they knew they had to make some changes.

So first they made absolutely sure that every dollar they spent . . . really hurt the dragon.

And that every hour they volunteered to fight against diabetes . . . really hurt the dragon.

And that the only experts they supported were people they could count on to . . . really hurt the dragon.

And THEN . . . they added the "secret ingredient."

And suddenly the sky turned black.

And the earth shook.

And the dragon gave a horrible moan.

He lashed out with his tail.

And his fire went out.

And finally he rolled over with his feet in the air.

And he died.

Hallelujah!

The Dragon Diabetes was dead!

And all the people danced for joy.

At last, just like all the other dinosaurs, the Diabetes Dragon had become EXTINCT.

He was gone forever . . . and the PEOPLE had done the job.

All there was left of diabetes was a rack of old bones in the Smithsonian Museum.

*   *   *

(. . . and by now, I'm sure you have guessed, the "secret ingredient" . . . is YOU!)

Reprinted with permission of Joan Hoover.

Doctor's Initial Examination

On your first visit to a new doctor or shortly thereafter, you should undergo a comprehensive evaluation of your diabetes. The following components are an indispensable part of that evaluation.

Complete History and Physical Examination

Although the history is probably the most important feature of the initial evaluation, full details cannot be provided here for space reasons. Essential points that should be covered include family history of diabetes; circumstances at the onset of the diabetes; history of treatment through diet, exercise, pills, and insulin; and evaluation of the effectiveness of current treatment. In addition, the presence of or potential for diabetic complications should also be reviewed. These complications are macrovascular (arteriosclerosis affecting circulation to the heart, legs, and brain); microvascular (affecting the retina and kidney); and neuropathic (leading to numbness in the feet, impotence, or other symptoms).

The physical exam should be as comprehensive as any you've ever had. Important aspects of the exam include:

- *Blood pressure.* A risk factor for diabetic complications and a reflection of subtle changes in kidney function.

- *Eyes.* Retinal exam to check for diabetic retinopathy.

- *Neck.* Evaluation for autoimmune thyroid disease.

- *Heart.* Check for macrovascular complications (arteriosclerosis) affecting circulation to the heart.

- *Pulse.* Evaluation for arteriosclerosis. Pulse should be checked in the neck, wrists, groin, top of foot, and inner ankle.

- *Neurological.* Check for sensations in the feet. "Reflexes" checked with a hammer tap at the ankle and knee.

- *Feet.* Examination for pulse and neurological function as well as deformities such as bunions or hammer toes, calluses, breaks in the skin, and improperly cut toenails.

Laboratory Evaluation

The following tests are especially important in evaluating a patient with diabetes:

- *Blood sugar.* A seemingly indispensable part of diabetes care, but is *one* blood sugar value really that important, compared with what the patient can test at home?

- *Glycosylated hemoglobin.* Essential in evaluating overall diabetes control and as a baseline for further improvements in therapy.

- *Cholesterol, HDL Cholesterol, triglycerides.* Total cholesterol and LDL Cholesterol (calculated from the three lipid tests) are used to evaluate the risk of diabetic macrovascular complications. Triglyceride values (which are often elevated in diabetes) may also reflect the level of overall diabetes control.

- *Creatinine.* A measure of kidney function, not especially sensitive to early changes. Measuring "creatinine clearance" by obtaining both a blood test and a twenty-four-hour urine specimen is much more sensitive.

■ *Urinalysis.* Important as a screen for infection and to look for urine protein.

■ *Microalbuminuria.* The most sensitive measure for early diabetes kidney effect, this test should become the standard for patients with diabetes. It can be measured with a random, overnight, or twenty-four-hour urine collection.

■ *Urine culture.* Should be done if the urinalysis shows any abnormality.

■ *Thyroid function tests.* Essential for every patient with Type I diabetes to be screened for autoimmune thyroid disease.

■ *Electrocardiogram (EKG).* Should be done routinely in patients who are over forty or who have had at least ten years of diabetes. A baseline reading is often done on all patients at the first visit.

These data form the basis of your initial evaluation and, in a shortened version, may become the model for a yearly diabetes update. But remember—medical care cannot be evaluated by a checklist; your own physician may have a different way of organizing the above data. Still, one way or another, this information should be part of every diabetic patient's record. Knowing what to expect, and what data to ask for, will help you become more informed about your own health and medical care.

Recommended Reading

. . . .

Basic Books on Diabetes

Anderson, James, M.D. *Diabetes: A Practical New Guide to Healthy Living.* New York: Warner Books, 1981. This book explains Dr. Anderson's High Carbohydrate-Fiber Nutrition plan (HCF), which he began developing in 1974. His diet is particularly helpful for overweight Type II's, as it features very low-fat meals. It lowers blood glucose, weight, and cholesterol. Dr. Anderson was one of the original oat bran enthusiasts and contributed much research for lowering cholesterol with fiber.

Biermann, June, and Barbara Toohey. *The Diabetic's Total Health Book.* 3rd. edition. Los Angeles: Jeremy P. Tarcher, 1992. The book that proves you can have a chronic disease and yet be the picture of health, leading a vital, productive, and happy life. It shows you how to do this by focusing on your health rather than on your disease. Teaches you how to achieve a strong body, a tranquil mind, and a blithe spirit. There are entertaining and effective sections on reducing stress and raising your spirits with travel, laughter, and hugs. The new edition is thoroughly up-to-date to reflect the latest changes in diabetes therapy and features thirty-five of June and Barbara's personal favorite recipes.

_____. *The Peripatetic Diabetic.* Revised edition. Los Angeles: Jeremy P. Tarcher, 1984. Originally published in 1969, this is June and Barbara's first and most personal diabetes book, the one that tells how to overcome that initial fear and despair and move on to a more joyful, exciting, and healthy life than ever before. This edition was updated to bring you into the contemporary world of diabetes therapy. But the original book with all of its crises and confusions is still there, exactly as it was written—and lived.

Curtis, Judy. *Living with Diabetic Complications.* Shippensburg, PA: Companion Press, 1993. This is a book about, for, and by people who are living with serious diabetic complications. It is full of sound, workable strategies for coping physically and emotionally and is very thorough on medical treatment options and sources of additional specialized help. The author has had Type I diabetes for forty-two years and has experienced vision impairment, kidney disease, heart disease, neuropathy, and an amputation. As part of her research, she sent out a questionnaire to hundreds of people with complications. Their responses and ideas connect this book with the reality of every kind of complications problem.

Etzwiler, Donnell D., M.D., ed., and others. *Learning to Live Well with Diabetes.* Revised edition. Minneapolis: International Diabetes Center, 1991. This is a very readable, easy-to-use comprehensive manual on managing diabetes written by over twenty-five prominent experts. It reflects the latest medical advances, technologies and research. There are over thirty chapters covering all aspects of self-care.

Guthrie, Diana, R.N., C.D.E., Ph.D., and Richard A. Guthrie, M.D. *The Diabetes Sourcebook.* Los Angeles: Lowell House, 1990. This is a basic reference guide by a renowned husband and wife nurse and doctor team. Always in the forefront of diabetes therapy and education, they here present information on how to give yourself the best care. Very good on interacting with health professionals and family and friends.

Jovanovic-Peterson, Lois, M.D., June Biermann, and Barbara Toohey. *The Diabetic Woman.* Los Angeles: Lowell House, 1987. The only book to focus on how women can deal with diabetes-related problems at the different ages of their lives. Here is medical advice and support and understanding as well as realistic coping methods for the complex concerns of today's woman. Dr. Jovanovic-

Peterson, Senior Scientist at Sansum Medical Research Foundation, in Santa Barbara, CA, is a diabetic and a wife and mother.

Krall, Leo P., M.D., and Richard S. Beaser, M.D. *Joslin Diabetes Manual.* 12th edition. Philadelphia: Lea and Febiger, 1989. Universally considered the Bible of Diabetes. This should be the cornerstone of everyone's diabetes reference library. All 406 pages are packed with the kind of information that will help you earn a Joslin Medal for fifty years of complication-free diabetes. The Joslin Clinic in Boston, opened in 1898, is the oldest diabetes treatment center in the United States.

Lodewick, Peter A., M.D., June Biermann, and Barbara Toohey. *The Diabetic Man.* Los Angeles: Lowell House, 1991. The guide to health and success in all areas of a man's life: career, sports, travel, dining, sex, relationships—everything. Includes a section with advice, empathy, and support for those with a diabetic man in their lives and for parents of a diabetic son. Dr. Lodewick is an endocrinologist, sportsman, and a well-controlled diabetic.

Lowe, Ernest, and Gary Arsham, M.D., Ph.D. *Diabetes: A Guide to Living Well.* 2nd Revised edition. Minneapolis: Chronimed Publishing, 1992. A management guide for Type I's, written by two authors who've had diabetes for more than thirty-five years, plus a special chapter for women by Kathy Feste, diabetic for over thirty years. The only book that gives individualized guidance in the sense that you're offered three programs of self-care: intensive, moderate, or loose. This is an all-inclusive book of concrete advice.

Milchovich, Sue K., R.N., C.D.E., and Barbara Dunn-Long, R.D. *Diabetes Mellitus: A Practical Handbook.* 5th Revised edition. Palo Alto, CA: Bull Publishing Company, 1992. This is an easy-to-use and thorough explanation of diabetes and how to control it. It is very complete on diet and food choices and includes the entire Exchange Lists and sample meals plans for different calorie levels. Large type. A good beginning book.

Peterson, Charles, M.D., and Lois Jovanovic-Peterson, M.D. *The Diabetes Self-Care Method.* Los Angeles: Lowell House, 1990. This book was written by two of the foremost endocrinologists of the U.S. before the DCCT study, but they had already foreseen the advantages of the intensive therapy approach. This is a best-selling, state-of-the-art manual which focuses on normalizing blood sugar through self-testing and insulin adjustment.

Type II Diabetes

Bernstein, Richard K., M.D., *Diabetes: Type II*. New York: Prentice-Hall Press, 1990. Dr. Bernstein, who has had Type I diabetes for forty-six years, worked out this very special regimen of meticulous control of blood sugar years ago. He believed in intensive therapy long, long before the DCCT study, which has proven him correct. His program is not easy, because the diet favors protein rather than carbohydrate foods. But his system does normalize blood sugar for those willing to adopt his methods. Also, the information in his previous book, *The GlucoGraf Method for Normalizing Blood Sugar* (1983), is updated for Type I's.

Monk, Arlene, R.D., C.D.E., and others. *Managing Type II Diabetes*. Wayzata, MN: DCI Publishing, 1988. This book is one of the first and best to deal exclusively with Type II diabetes. Thirty chapters written by twenty-four prominent health-care experts of the International Diabetes Center. It gives a complete understanding of the special problems of Type II's and tells the steps to take to handle them.

Valentine, Virginia, R.N., M.S., C.D.E., June Biermann, and Barbara Toohey. *Diabetes Type II and What to Do*. Los Angeles: Lowell House, 1993. This latest and most-up-to-date book on Type II is accurate, practical, and, above all, compassionate. Its ongoing message is "Type II Diabetes Is Not a Character Flaw." Virginia Valentine, herself Type II, clearly explains the difference between those who are overweight and have insulin resistance (Type II-R) and those who are of normal weight but are deficient in insulin (Type II-D). Entertaining and packed with information. Type II's will love it, and, more important, it will make them love and care for themselves.

Emotional Health and Stress

Edelwich, Jerry, and Archie Brodsky. *Diabetes: Caring for Your Emotions.* New York: Addison-Wesley, 1986. This book explores the deepest feelings of diabetics. It is told in the words of the people who lived through them. Outstanding chapters on sexuality, conflicts with health professionals, and family dynamics. Type II diabetics, who often get short shrift, are given as much attention as Type I's.

Rubin, Richard R., Ph.D., June Biermann, and Barbara Toohey. *Psyching Out Diabetes: A Positive Approach to Your Negative Emotions.* Los Angeles: Lowell House, 1992. Diabetes control can be 90 percent in your head. This exciting, breakthrough book helps you straighten out your head and get rid of the fear, denial, depression, grief, frustration, embarrassment, and guilt that block good diabetes control and a good life. Shows how to improve your perspective and enables you to look at your diabetic challenges in a completely different way. Dr. Rubin is on the faculty of the Johns Hopkins Medical School and has a private practice in Baltimore. He has counseled diabetic patients for over twenty years and has a diabetic son and sister. Dr. Rubin speaks clearly, directly, and without any psychological mumbo-jumbo.

Parents and Children

Betschart, Jean, M.N., R.N., C.D.E. *It's Time to Learn About Diabetes.* Minneapolis: DCI Publishing, 1991. This workbook on diabetes for children ages eight to ten years is creatively and professionally written by a highly experienced Certified Diabetes Educator of the Children's Hospital of Pittsburgh. Will truly help any child (or parent!) learn good diabetes self-care. Wonderfully illustrated. Fill-in quizzes for each chapter. A uniquely important book for home and diabetes education class use. Invaluable for the newly diagnosed child.

Folkman, Jane, R.D., and Hugo Hollerorth, Ed. D. *A Guide for Women with Diabetes Who Are Pregnant or Plan to Be.* Boston: Joslin Diabetes Center, 1986. Produced at the Pregnancy Clinic of the renowned Joslin Diabetes Center, this clearly written labor of love includes everything learned at the nation's first diabetes clinic to care for the distinctive needs of pregnant women with diabetes. The most complete manual available on the subject.

Heegard, Marge, M.A., and Chris Ternand, M.D. *When a Family Gets Diabetes.* Minneapolis: DCI Publishing, 1990. This book uses art therapy to help children with diabetes and their families understand and express their feelings about the disease. The child and family members draw pictures that relate to certain aspects of diabetes and then discuss why they drew what they did. An excellent communication tool.

Johnson, Robert Wood, IV, Sale Johnson, Casey Johnson, and Susan Kleinman. *Managing Your Child's Diabetes.* New York: MasterMedia Limited, 1992. This book, written by a father, mother, and diabetic daughter, is a boon for parents of newly diagnosed children. The first chapter, by Casey Johnson, who was diagnosed at age eight, was written when she was twelve and is a little masterpiece of advice to all parents. The rest of the book is detailed information on blood-sugar control as well as how to deal with doctors and hospitals, teachers and schools, and the rest of the diabetic child's family. The last chapter, by Kenneth Farber, executive director of the Juvenile Diabetes Foundation International, is an encouraging look into the future.

Loring, Gloria. *Parenting a Diabetic Child.* Los Angeles: Lowell House, 1993. This TV star and celebrity chairman of the Juvenile Diabetes Foundation has parented her diabetic son for over twelve years. This is a complex job, requiring expert technical information, psychological insight, and emotional support. Gloria provides all three for parents of diabetic children, leading you gently and authoritatively as only a mother who's been there can.

Roberts, Willo Davis. *Sugar Isn't Everything.* New York: Macmillan, 1987. The subtitle of this novel is *A Support Book, in Fiction Form, for the Young Diabetic.* A professional children's book writer who herself became diabetic as an adult, Willo Roberts turned her own new knowledge and experience into a factually sound, therapeutically up-to-date novel with an eleven-year-old girl as its heroine. Amy develops diabetes, struggles with it, learns how to handle it, and eventually accepts it. Engrossing and true to life. Every young diabetic can relate to this novel, and learn more and feel better for having read it. Good for parents, too.

Cookbooks, Nutrition, Weight Loss, and Exchanges

ADA Family Cookbooks. 4 vols. New York: Prentice-Hall, Vols. I–III 1987, Vol. IV 1991. These four cookbooks are healthy eating guides for the entire family, not just for the diabetic members. Vol. I has 250 recipes, information on nutrition, meal planning, exchanges, dining out, and fast food. Vol. II has 206 recipes, four chapters on fighting fat, an exercise program, ethnic dishes and exchanges plus a section on fiber. Vol. III focuses on variety and popular ethnic dishes such as tortilla soup, fajitas, and jambalaya. Features quick-cooking tips; microwaving method included when appropriate. All recipes reduced in fat, low in sodium, and limited to a half teaspoon of sugar. Vol. IV features the rich, traditional recipes from every region of America—the foods everyone loves best.

Cooper, Nancy, R.D. *The Joy of Snacks.* Minneapolis: Chronimed, 1991. For Type II's, snacking six to ten times a day is actually better than eating three square meals. Type I's need handy snacks to prevent or treat low-blood-sugar episodes. Here's a book, written by an acclaimed dietitian, to help both types. Lots of muffin and cookie recipes and a large selection of popcorn treats and special snacks for kids. Two hundred delicious recipes with exchanges.

Finsand, Mary Jane. *The Complete Diabetic Cookbook.* New York: Sterling Publishing Company, 1987. Everything from snacks to sophisticated gourmet dishes packed into one slim volume. Includes ADA exchanges. Real food that is simple to prepare.

———. *Diabetic Cakes, Pies, & Other Scrumptious Desserts.* New York: Sterling Publishing Company, 1988. Another treasury of 200 formerly forbidden delights for people with diabetes and weight watchers. Even includes a Grand Marnier soufflé! Gives exchanges and calorie and carbohydrate counts.

———. *The Diabetic Candy, Cookie, and Dessert Cookbook.* New York: Sterling Publishing Company, 1982. Chemist-nutritionist Finsand gives you over two hundred recipes using sugar replacements. A treasure of thrills for dessertees. Even tells you how to make ice-cream cones. Contains twelve pie recipes, seventeen cake recipes, and forty-four cookie recipes.

———. *The Diabetic Chocolate Cookbook.* New York: Sterling Publishing Company, 1984. The luxury of chocolate in candies, cookies, cakes, pies, and puddings is here made possible for diabetics. Exchanges and calories are provided for each recipe.

———. *Diabetic Microwave Cookbook.* New York: Sterling Publishing Company, 1989. Almost 300 recipes covering an amazing array of dining choices, with emphasis on protein dishes, all prepared quickly, easily, and healthily in a microwave.

———. *Quick and Delicious Diabetic Desserts.* New York: Sterling Publishing Company, 1992. Scores of recipes for pies and puddings, cakes and cookies, ice creams and tortes. Luscious treats that will augment any meal.

Franz, Marion, M.S., R.D. *Exchanges for All Occasions.* Minneapolis: Chronimed, 1993. Packed full of sound, authoritative guidance for diabetic eating. This new edition has the latest nutrition facts and recommendations, even the new Food Guide Pyramid and labeling system. Lists hundreds of foods not on the ADA exchange lists. Covers every eating situation (camping, children's parties, holidays) and most cuisines (Jewish, Southwestern, vegetarian, etc.).

Gilliard, Judy, and J. Kirkpatrick. *Guiltless Gourmet.* Wayzata, Minn.: Diabetes Center, Inc., 1987. By a dietitian and a diabetic trained in classic French cuisine. This book has sophisticated recipes from all over the world, all computer analyzed for the diabetic diet. All are low in fat, cholesterol, sugar, and calories.

Hess, Mary Abbott, R.D., M.S., and Katherine Middleton. Chicago: Contemporary Books, 1988. This could be called the diabetic person's *Joy of Cooking* because it has everything you need to know to understand the diet, plan and prepare delicious meals and snacks, and love doing it! Nondiabetics who share the meals won't believe they're on the diabetic diet. Contains 350 recipes that are low in saturated fats and sugar.

Kruppa, Carole. *Free and Equal Cookbook.* Chicago: Surrey Books, 1988. The original, highly popular cookbook featuring all recipes with Equal (NutraSweet). The author grew up in a French family and does not sacrifice good taste in these 150 low-calorie and sugar-free recipes. Includes breakfast treats, appetizers, soups, salads, entrees, desserts, beverages, and jams. Gives calorie counts and exchanges for all recipes.

_____. *Free and Equal Dessert Cookbook.* Chicago: Surrey Books, 1992. One hundred and fifty quick and delicious low-calorie desserts and sweet treats all using the sweetener Equal (NutraSweet). All recipes are also low-salt and low-cholesterol. Includes exchanges and calories.

Majors, Judith S. *Sugar Free Good and Easy; Sugar Free Goodies; Sugar Free Kids' Cookery.* Milwaukie, Ore.: Apple Press, 1987, 1987, 1989. Finally back in print, three books approved by the Oregon affiliate of the ADA and written by a diabetic woman who confesses she "lives to eat." All recipes are simple and quick. *Goodies* is for those with a sweet tooth—pies, cookies, jams, ice creams. *Good and Easy* has breads, salads, main dishes— everything for variety and good meals. *Kids' Cookery* has recipes with child appeal that are simple enough for young diabetics to prepare. Exchanges in each book.

Marks, Betty. *Microwave Diabetic Cookbook.* Chicago: Surrey Books, 1991. Over 130 fast, sugar-free recipes, all high in taste but low in fat, cholesterol, sodium, and calories. You can make a delicious meal in fifteen minutes or less thanks to the busy author, who is a literary agent, a prizewinning ballroom dancer, and an insulin-dependent person with diabetes.

Natow, Annette, Ph.D., R.D., and Jo Ann Heslin, R.D. *Diabetes Carbohydrate and Calorie Counter.* New York: Pocket Books, 1991. Gives carbohydrate, calorie, and fat count in grams for 3,000 foods from Abalone to Zucchini. Includes takeout and frozen items. Excellent guidelines for designing an eating plan for Type II diabetes.

————. *The Fat Counter.* New York: Pocket Books, 1993. Fat is the enemy of health; fat is the particular enemy of people with diabetes, especially Type II's. Among other things, it interferes with the action of insulin. This handy book gives the data needed to learn how to avoid it. Fat and calorie values given for over 10,000 foods, including packaged and frozen foods, thirty-six fast food chains, and prepared recipes and snacks. A Bible of healthy avoidance.

Robertson, Laurel, Carol Flinders, and Brian Ruppenthal. *The New Laurel's Kitchen.* Berkeley: Ten Speed Press, 1986. *Laurel's Kitchen* has always been our favorite vegetarian cookbook. The new *Laurel* has the same inspiring philosophy and new recipes that open vistas of dining joy and health. Tells how to increase fiber and cut back on fat. Sections on cooking for children, elders, pregnant women, and athletes. Also now available in the abridged version: *Laurel's Kitchen Recipes.*

Schneider, Clara G., R.D. *Diabetic's Brand Name Food Exchange Handbook,* Philadelphia: Running Press, 1991. The second revised and expanded edition of the best-selling essential guide to supermarket shopping and fast-food dining. Gives exchanges, calorie counts, and sodium values for nearly 4,000 brand-name foods and snacks, including frozen dinners, baby foods, lunch meats, fast foods, alcoholic beverages, and sugar-free snacks.

Shaevitz, Morton H., Ph.D. *Lean and Mean: The No-Hassle, Life-Extending Weight Loss Program for Men.* New York: Putnam, 1993. Sound, easy-to-follow advice for men who don't like how they feel and look and who want to do something about it now. (But who don't want weight loss to be the prime focus of their lives!) Excellent for overweight Type II men. Includes a section for the women who love them and want to help them lose weight without nagging. Tips are equally valid for career women who have to try to lose weight while fulfilling all of their social and business obligations.

Warshaw, Hope S., M.M.Sc. *The Restaurant Companion.* Chicago: Surrey Books, 1990. The first book to focus entirely on restaurant dining. Shows how to make appropriate healthy choices for eight ethnic cuisines, including Mexican, Chinese, Italian, and Thai, as well as for American and fast-food restaurants. Also gives advice for salad bars, brunches, and airline meals. Describes ingredients in typical dishes and gives exchanges for recommended choices.

Waterhouse, Debra, M.P.H., R.D. *Outsmarting the Female Fat Cell.* New York: Hyperion, 1993. The first weight-control program specifically designed for women. Based on scientific data and the author's experiences in her private practice as a registered dietitian. Designed to get women's fat cells to burn, not store fat. Shows how to stop starving and start eating by fatproofing your diet. Includes this sound advice: find your comfortable and healthy weight that is not determined by society but by your body type and genetics.

Exercise

Bailey, Covert. *The New Fit of Fat.* Boston: Houghton Mifflin, 1991. The essential message of this well-researched breakthrough book is that overweight people should concentrate on losing body fat, not pounds. Bailey says that fat people often eat less than skinny people and the only way they can lose body fat is through exercise that changes their metabolism. Exercise resets all the body mechanisms to lower body fat. His message: "The ultimate cure for obesity is exercise." Other valuable books for following Bailey's program are *Fit or Fat Target Diet* and *Fit or Fat Target Recipes.*

Franz, Marion J., M.S., R.D., and Jane Norstrom, M.A. *Diabetes: Actively Staying Healthy.* Minneapolis: DCI. A well-rounded, fact-filled guide to devising a game plan to use exercise as the cornerstone of diabetes treatment and general fitness. Broad coverage:

beginner's programs, tips for Type I's and Type II's, diabetic athletes, and three chapters on fuel metabolism for those who want to
have an in-depth understanding of what goes on in the body during
exercise. Many tables and charts.

Gordon, Neil F., M.D., Ph.D., M.P.H. *Diabetes: Your Complete Exercise Guide.* Champaign: Human Kinetics, 1993. Shows how a
regular exercise program combined with proper nutrition and medication can help people with diabetes control their disease and improve their health. Describes the exercises and activities that are
most beneficial for increasing flexibility, strength, and aerobic fitness as well as reducing the risk of complications.

Magazines

Countdown, 432 Park Avenue South, New York, NY 10016-8013
(1-800-223-1138). The magazine of the Juvenile Diabetes Foundation International. Published four times a year. Subscription
price $25.

Diabetes Forecast, the magazine of the American Diabetes Association, 1660 Duke St., Alexandria, VA 22314 (1-800-232-3472).
Published monthly. Membership dues are $24 per year, $10 of
which is designated for the subscription.

Diabetes in the News, Ames Center for Diabetes Education, Miles,
Inc., Diagnostics Division, 224 E. Monroe, South Bend, IN 46601
(312-664-9782). Provides useful information to help people with
diabetes improve their lives. Published bimonthly. Subscription
price $12. (Address subscriptions to P.O. Box 4548, South Bend,
IN 46634.)

Diabetes Interview, 3715 Balboa Street, San Francisco, CA 94121
(415-387-4002). A consumer-oriented newspaper for the diabetes
community, includes reports on current research, business briefs,
articles. Published monthly. Subscription price $14.

The Diabetic Reader, June & Barbara, Ink/Prana Publications, 5623
Matilija Ave., Van Nuys, CA 91401 (1-800-735-7726). Reviews and

excerpts latest books on diabetes, includes offbeat feature articles on living the good life with diabetes, catalog of available diabetes books. Published sporadically. Free.

The Diabetic Traveler, P.O. Box 8223 RW, Stamford, CT 06905. A newsletter focusing on practical information to encourage people with diabetes to live—and travel—as normally as possible. Published quarterly. $18.95.

Index